T0226990

Cosmetic Dermatology for Men

Editor

NEIL S. SADICK

DERMATOLOGIC CLINICS

www.derm.theclinics.com

Consulting Editor
BRUCE H. THIERS

January 2018 • Volume 36 • Number 1

ELSEVIER

1600 John F. Kennedy Boulevard • Suite 1800 • Philadelphia, Pennsylvania, 19103-2899

http://www.theclinics.com

DERMATOLOGIC CLINICS Volume 36, Number 1
January 2018 ISSN 0733-8635, ISBN-13: 978-0-323-56637-7

Editor: Jessica McCool
Developmental Editor: Sara Watkins

Dermatologic Clinics (ISSN 0733-8635) is published quarterly by Elsevier Inc., 360 Park Avenue South, New York, NY 10010-1710. Months of publication are January, April, July, and October. Business and editorial offices: 1600 John F. Kennedy Blvd., Suite 1800, Philadelphia, PA 19103-2899. Customer service office: 11830 Westline Drive, St. Louis, MO 63146. Periodicals postage paid at New York, NY, and additional mailing offices. Subscription prices are USD 392.00 per year for US individuals, USD 701.00 per year for US institutions, USD 451.00 per year for Canadian individuals, USD 855.00 per year for Canadian institutions, USD 505.00 per year for international individuals, USD 855.00 per year for international institutions, USD 100.00 per year for US students/residents, and USD 240.00 per year for Canadian and international students/residents. International air speed delivery is included in all *Clinics* subscription prices. All prices are subject to change without notice. **POSTMASTER:** Send address changes to *Dermatologic Clinics*, Elsevier Health Sciences Division, Subscription Customer Service, 3251 Riverport Lane, Maryland Heights, MO 63043. **Customer Service: 1-800-654-2452 (U.S. and Canada); 314-447-8871 (outside U.S. and Canada). Fax: 314-447-8029. E-mail: journalscustomerservice-usa@elsevier.com (for print support); journalsonlinesupport-usa@elsevier.com (for online support).**

Reprints. For copies of 100 or more, of articles in this publication, please contact the Commercial Reprints Department, Elsevier Inc., 360 Park Avenue South, New York, New York 10010-1710. Tel.: 212-633-3874; Fax: 212-633-3820; Email: reprints@elsevier.com.

The *Dermatologic Clinics* is covered in *MEDLINE/PubMed (Index Medicus)*, *Current Contents/Clinical Medicine*, *Excerpta Medica*, *Chemical Abstracts*, and *ISI/BIOMED*.

Contributors

CONSULTING EDITOR

BRUCE H. THIERS, MD
Professor and Chairman Emeritus, Department
of Dermatology and Dermatologic Surgery,
Medical University of South Carolina,
Charleston, South Carolina, USA

EDITOR

**NEIL S. SADICK, MD, FACP, FAACS, FACPh,
FAAD**
Clinical Professor, Department of
Dermatology, Weill Cornell Medicine, New
York, New York, USA; Associate Director of
Clinical Research, Co-Director of Aesthetics
Education, Department of Dermatology,
University of Buffalo, Buffalo, New York, USA

AUTHORS

ZOE DIANA DRAELOS, MD
Consulting Professor, Department of
Dermatology, Duke University School of
Medicine, Durham, North Carolina, USA;
Private Practice, Dermatology Consulting
Services, High Point, North Carolina, USA

SABRINA G. FABI, MD
Dermatologist, Cosmetic Laser Dermatology,
Goldman, Butterwick, Groff, Fabi, and Wu,
a West Dermatology Company, Assistant
Professor, Department of Dermatology,
University of California San Diego, San Diego,
California, USA

MICHAEL H. GOLD, MD
Visiting Professor of The People's Hospital of
Hunan Province, Medical Director, Gold Skin
Care Center, Tennessee Clinical Research
Center, Assistant Clinical Professor, Vanderbilt
University School of Nursing, Adjunct Assistant
Professor, Meharry Medical College, School of
Medicine, Nashville, Tennessee, USA;

Physician Assistant Student Preceptor, Wake
Forest School of Medicine, Winston-Salem,
North Carolina, USA; Visiting Professor of
Dermatology, Huashan Hospital, Fudan
University, Shanghai, China; First Hospital of
China Medical University, Shenyang, China;
Guangdong Provincial People's Hospital,
Visiting Professor of Plastic Surgery, First
People's Hospital of Foshan, Guangzhou,
China; Zhejiang University, Hangzhou,
Zhejiang, China; Visiting Professor, Rongjun
Hospital, Jiaxing, China

DAVID J. GOLDBERG, MD, JD
Private Practice, Skin Laser & Surgery
Specialists, Clinical Professor, Dermatology,
Icahn School of Medicine at Mount Sinai,
Adjunct Professor, Law, Fordham University
School of Law, New York, New York, USA; Skin
Laser & Surgery Specialists, Hackensack, New
Jersey, USA; Clinical Professor, Dermatology,
Rutgers New Jersey Medical School, Newark,
New Jersey, USA

Contributors

MITCHEL P. GOLDMAN, MD
Private Practice, Goldman, Butterwick, Groff, Fabi, and Wu Cosmetic Laser Dermatology, San Diego, California, USA

MARC ZACHARY HANDLER, MD
Private Practice, Skin Laser & Surgery Specialists, New York, New York, USA; Skin Laser & Surgery Specialists, Hackensack, New Jersey; Dermatology, Rutgers New Jersey Medical School, Newark, New Jersey, USA

MICHELLE HENRY, MD
Clinical Instructor, Department of Dermatology, Weill Cornell Medicine, New York, New York, USA

ISABELA T. JONES, MD
Dermatologist, McLean Dermatology and Skincare Center, McLean, Virginia, USA

MARGIT JUHÁSZ, MD
Marmur Medical, New York, New York, USA; Department of Dermatology, University of California, Irvine, Irvine, California, USA

CHERYL KARCHER, MD
Department of Dermatology, Weill Cornell Medicine, Sadick Dermatology, New York, New York, USA

ELLEN MARMUR, MD
Marmur Medical, Department of Dermatology, Mount Sinai Hospital, New York, New York, USA

PAUL T. ROSE, MD, FAAD, JD
Coral Gables, Florida, USA

NEIL S. SADICK, MD, FACP, FAACS, FACPh, FAAD
Clinical Professor, Department of Dermatology, Weill Cornell Medicine, New York, New York, USA; Associate Director of Clinical Research, Co-Director of Aesthetics Education, Department of Dermatology, University of Buffalo, Buffalo, New York, USA

HEIDI WAT, MD
Division of Dermatology, Department of Medicine, University of Alberta, Edmonton, Alberta, Canada

DOUGLAS C. WU, MD, PhD
Private Practice, Goldman, Butterwick, Groff, Fabi, and Wu Cosmetic Laser Dermatology, San Diego, California, USA

Contents

Increasing numbers of men are seeking aesthetic treatments for fat reduction, skin rejuvenation, and other antiaging goals. Compared with women, however, men have distinctly different anatomy and physiologic differences that manifest in the aging process. Given that both anatomy and the aging process affect treatment strategies and clinical outcomes, there is a need for dermatologists to be acutely aware of these male-specific nuances to provide the best clinical care and patient satisfaction.

Men are interested in reducing signs of aging, while maintaining a masculine appearance. A chief concern among men is maintenance of scalp hair. Men are also concerned with reducing under eye bags and dark circles. The concern of feminization is of significant importance. Neuromodulators remain the most common cosmetic procedure performed in men. Men often prefer a reduction in facial rhytids, as opposed to elimination of the lines. Softening facial lines in men is meant to maintain an appearance of wisdom, without appearing fragile. Men also wish to maintain a taut jawline and a slim waist and reduce breast tissue.

Men of all races are currently more open to requesting and undergoing treatments for a plethora of cosmetic concerns. Among the most common goals are procedures that combat the signs of aging, rejuvenate the skin, even out the color tone, address textural issues such as acne scarring, and improve hair disorders. Given the differences in cultural ideals and anatomic/physiologic differences in ethnic skin, it is important for physicians to be aware and sensitive to the nuances required when providing consultation and treating non-Caucasian men. The main cosmetic concerns of this patient cohort and their optimal management are presented.

The male cosmeceutical market is still underdeveloped. Although women embrace skin care as a part of general health, this concept has not gained wide male acceptance. Shaving is probably the most beneficial daily grooming event men commonly undertake for skin appearance and may account for the failure of antiaging cosmeceuticals to attract attention in this segment. In addition, there are many physiologic differences between male and female skin, with less of a need for moisturization and photoprotection in men. This article highlights some of the differences between male and female skin along with the unique product attributes required to address these differences.

Men seek cosmetic procedures for vastly different reasons than women. Men often seek discrete cosmetic services with little downtime. Male skin structure generally differs from female skin structure. Dermatologists should consider subtle differences in the psyche of the male cosmetic patient.

Injection of neurotoxin is the most commonly performed cosmetic procedure in the United States, and the total number of male patients seeking botulinum has steadily increased over the years. Because of their unique aesthetic goals, expectations, and anatomy, men require differing botulinum toxin doses and techniques. This article provides an evidence-based approach to botulinum toxin in men. Each area of the face is discussed separately, focusing on gender differences in anatomy, treatment goals, and injection method.

Fillers and toxins are safe, quick, and require no downtime; the immediately visible results can boost a man's self-esteem, confidence, youthfulness, and sense of competitiveness in the personal and professional realms of the world. The approach to using these agents has changed from ironing out the skin to remove wrinkles and lines to a restructuring of the 3-dimensional face. This new strategy, volumetric structural rejuvenation (VSR), relies on intimate knowledge of facial anatomy and the pathophysiology of aging. It is of essence to know the key anatomic differences between the 2 sexes to avoid potential feminization.

Noninvasive body contouring is an attractive therapeutic modality to enhance the ideal male physique. Men place higher value on enhancing a well-defined, strong, masculine jawline and developing a V-shaped taper through the upper body. An understanding of the body contour men strive for allows the treating physician to focus on areas that are of most concern to men, thus enhancing patient experience and satisfaction. This article discusses noninvasive body contouring techniques, taking into account the unique aesthetic concerns of the male patient by combining an analysis of the existing literature with the authors' own clinical experience.

Hair loss affects millions of people worldwide and can have devastating effects on an individual's psychological and emotional well-being. Hair restoration technologies have advanced with the use of robotics and manual and motorized follicular unit extraction to provide patients excellent clinical results. Adjuvant modalities, such as platelet-rich plasma injections, lasers, and stem cells, can further enhance the survivability and appearance of hair transplants.

DERMATOLOGIC CLINICS

THE CLINICS ARE AVAILABLE ONLINE!
Access your subscription at:
www.theclinics.com

Preface
Cosmetic Dermatology for Men

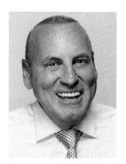

Neil S. Sadick, MD, FACP, FAACS, FACPh, FAAD
Editor

Today, men of all walks of life actively seek and embrace the benefits derived from undergoing aesthetic treatments. Aside from statistics reporting increased numbers of treatments performed on men, our personal experience is testament to this. In contrast to the past where most of our patients were women, today the numbers of female and male patients asking for cosmetic treatments are comparable. Despite this, physicians tend to not be attuned to the differences in treating the two genders; in fact, they tend to treat them in the same manner.

By default, male physiology, anatomy, and with exceptions, their general behavioral tendencies are different than women in ways that impact treatment. In addition, men's goals and motivation for aesthetic procedures are different. While women want to be young and beautiful, men simply desire to improve their appearance. They want to appear relaxed and youthful in society, and particularly competitive in their workplace.

The aim of this supplement is to guide both novice and experienced dermatologic surgeons to all aspects that impact treating their male patients. The different articles within this issue are written from the perspectives of plastic surgeons and dermatologists with the ultimate goal of increasing positive clinical outcomes and the satisfaction of their male patients. This collaborative effort has resulted in a comprehensive supplement that provides practical, up-to-date tips that physicians can use in their day-to-day treatment of men. Moreover, a scientific review of the current landscape is also incorporated in each article to bolster practical approaches with the latest available clinical research.

The subjects that the authors have included span from describing the basic pathophysiology of aging in men to the specifics of male liposuction. Drs Goldberg and Handler review cosmetic concerns in men, while Dr Henry focuses on aesthetic treatments pertinent to ethnic men. Dr Draelos and Drs Marmur and Juhász review male cosmeceutical skincare options and energy-based devices for skin rejuvenation, respectively. The importance of treating men with neurotoxins in a different

Dermatol Clin 36 (2018) ix–x
https://doi.org/10.1016/j.det.2017.09.011
0733-8635/18/© 2017 Published by Elsevier Inc.

manner than that done in women, to avoid feminization, is elaborated on by Drs Fabi and Jones. I also describe my methodology to volumetrically structurally rejuvenate the male face with new generation fillers. Drs Goldman, Wat, and Wu discuss noninvasive body contouring options for the upper and lower body, and Dr Gold presents combination strategies that men can take advantage of to maximize positive clinical outcomes. A big concern in men, hair loss, is also thoroughly discussed. Dr Rose focuses on hair transplantation, while I touch upon other nonsurgical hair loss treatments. Finally, Dr Karcher's article focuses on liposuction in men, one of the most popular surgical cosmetic procedures they ask for.

Our hope is that this supplement brings the male patient to the forefront of clinical research and care, so physicians can be intimately attuned to their needs and treat them accordingly.

Neil S. Sadick, MD, FACP, FAACS, FACPh, FAAD
Department of Dermatology
Weill Cornell Medicine
New York, NY 10065, USA

Department of Dermatology
University of Buffalo
Buffalo, NY 14260, USA

Sadick Dermatology
911 Park Avenue, Suite 1A
New York, NY 10075, USA

E-mail address:
nssderm@sadickdermatology.com

The Pathophysiology of the Male Aging Face and Body

Neil S. Sadick, MD[a,b,]*

KEYWORDS

- Aging • Pathophysiology • Men • Fat • Muscle • Skin

KEY POINTS

- The aging process in men is mainly driven by the differences in androgens.
- Male skin is thicker, muscle mass is greater, and subcutaneous adipose tissue is thinner than that of women.
- Men are less likely to engage in preventative measures to limit the effect of extrinsic factor in their aging process.

INTRODUCTION

Once a female-dominated field, today aesthetics and the pursuit of youth are high priorities for men of all ages, ethnicities, and cultures. From over-the-counter gender-specific cosmetics to in-office cosmetic treatments, men are taking their appearance more seriously than ever. According to the American Society for Aesthetic Plastic Surgery, the number of cosmetic procedures performed on men has increased more than 325% since 1997, and in 2015 alone, men had close to 1.2 million procedures, making up 10% of the total number of plastic surgeries performed for the year. Statistics also reveal that men tend to seek mostly minimally invasive procedures with little or no downtime; between 2010 and 2014, the use of botulinum toxin in men increased by 84%, hyaluronic acid fillers increased by 94%, and intense pulse light treatments increased by 44%.[1] Men and women are not created equal, however, when it comes to their motivations, goals, and their anatomy and relevant gender-specific pathophysiology that ultimately affect both treatment

strategy and clinical outcomes. For the practicing dermatologist who treats this increasing male patient demographic, intimate knowledge of both anatomic differences of the male face and body and the factors underlying the pathophysiology of aging is critical for delivering the best clinical results.

PATHOPHYSIOLOGY OF AGING IN MEN

Aging regardless of gender is characterized by progressive changes associated with increased susceptibility to many diseases and is influenced by intrinsic (genetic) and extrinsic factors (lifestyle choices and environmental exposures). A study in twins found that genetics accounted for approximately 25% of the variation in longevity, and although environmental factors accounted for approximately 50%, with greater longevity (to age 90 or 100), genetic influences became more important.[2] Several overarching physiologic principles characterize aging: loss of complexity as seen in less variability in heart rate responses, altered circadian patterns, loss of physiologic

Disclosure Statement: N. Sadick has nothing he wishes to disclose.
a Department of Dermatology, Weill Cornell Medicine, New York, NY, USA; b Department of Dermatology, University of Buffalo, Buffalo, NY, USA
* 911 Park Avenue, New York, NY 10075.
E-mail address: nssderm@sadickdermatology.com

derm.theclinics.com

reserves needed to cope with challenges to homeostasis and compromised immune function that contributes to increased frequency of infections, malignancies, and autoimmune disorders, ultimately leading to a chronic, low-level inflammatory state. In men, a key factor that contributes to the sexual dimorphism observed with aging is the decline of testosterone (as rapidly as 0.4%–2% annually after age 30 years). Because testosterone has a critical role in the modulation of adult male reproductive health, sexual function, bone health, fat metabolism, and muscle mass and strength, its declining levels have male-specific repercussions during the aging process.[3] Moreover, as opposed to women, who are equipped with innate antioxidant protection due to the presence of estrogen that mediates the expression of superoxide dismutase and other antioxidant molecules,[4] men are more susceptible to the action of free radicals and suffer from higher levels of oxidative stress.[5,6] These intrinsic factors together with the environment and lifestyle choices affect every organ system in men. Compared with women, men experience a steeper decline in pulmonary and aerobic function with age; studies have shown 3% to 6% decrease in peak aerobic capacity per decade in the 30s and more than 20% decrease in peak aerobic capacity per decade in the 70s and beyond.[7]

The effects of aging on the skin are the most revealing of a person's age, and studies have shown that men generally appear older than they actually are compared with women.[8] The male epidermis and dermis are thicker than those of women, with higher density of hair follicles, greater sebum and sweat production, and an increased ratio of muscle to subcutaneous tissue.[9,10] Due to the thicker skin and prominent facial musculature, the loss of subcutaneous adipose with age results in deeper expression lines in men compared with women, who typically develop superficial rhytides. Because androgen levels decline during aging, skin changes, with atrophy, decreased elasticity, and impaired metabolic and reparative responses the main manifestations. The epidermis becomes thinner and the dermoepidermal junction flattens, resulting in increased fragility of the skin to shear stress, decreased nutrient transfer, compromised skin barrier function of the skin, and redistribution of hair follicle.[11,12] As androgens convert vellus into terminal hairs, androgen-dependent areas (chin, upper lip, chest, breasts, abdomen, back, and anterior thighs) subsequently exhibit increased vascularity; as a result, decline of hormones during aging contributes to particular atrophy in those areas. Changes in the glycosaminoglycan macromolecules in the dermis lead to loss of hydration and decreased skin resilience and the decrease in subdermal fat. This loss of support contributes to the skin wrinkling and sagging as well as to increased susceptibility to trauma.[13]

As individuals age, muscle mass decreases in relation to body weight by approximately 30% to 50% in a nonlinear manner, that is, the loss is accelerated with advancing age. One major cause of this muscle mass loss is the decline of anabolic hormones, such as testosterone, dehydroepiandrosterone, and growth hormone, which results in a katabolic effect on muscles and bones.[14] Although men have significantly more skeletal, facial mimetic and fat-free muscle mass compared with women,[15] studies have reported a decreased muscle protein synthesis rate in older men compared with women with similar age/weight.[14] This decreased muscle function affects the male metabolism and lends susceptibility to increased accumulation to adipose tissue. Moreover, the loss of facial muscle mass and function with aging manifests in deep lines in men and a different wrinkle pattern.[16]

The proinflammatory environment together with the loss of minerals and change in hormones leads to increased probability of bone fractures and slower rate of repair, once fracture occurs. Bone loss has physical consequences in the face, because it provides the structural framework where soft tissues rest; men have prominent supraorbital ridges, greater glabellar projection, larger orbital size, and a wider chin contributing to the angular features of the aging male face.[17,18] With bone loss in the aging face, there is ptosis of tissues manifesting as undesirable sagging that motivates men for aesthetic interventions.

Fat mass and adipose tissue are also influenced by age in a gender-specific way. Body fat is redistributed and accumulates in the trunk and lower body while subcutaneous adipose tissue decreased.[19] Although men have less fat than women (10% to 15% in men compared with 18% and 20% in women of body weight), during aging its distributed more specifically in the abdominal region, lending susceptibility to cardiovascular disease and diabetes. In the face, men have a distinctly different adipose compartment distribution compared with women. The subcutaneous adipose layer is thinner overall and in areas, such as the malar areas, 3-D CT studies have demonstrated that men have less soft tissue and as much as 3 mm less subcutaneous tissue compared with women.[20,21] Moreover, the ratio of medial to lateral cheek thickness is 1.5:1 in women and 1.1:1, which clinically manifests as the flat and angular malar regions of men. In other facial regions, such as the orbital region, the orbital fat is larger compared with women, and depletion of the orbital fat pads with aging leads to lower eyelid prominence.[22]

Extrinsic factors, lifestyle choices, and environmental exposures accelerate the aging process. Prolonged and repeated exposure to solar radiation leads to premature skin aging, known as photoaging, that superimposed on the changes caused by chronologic aging is responsible for most of the age-associated features of skin appearance.[23] The mechanisms underlying the UV-mediated damage to the skin connective tissue involve the formation of reactive oxygen species (ROS), cell surface receptor-initiated signaling, protein oxidation, and mitochondrial damage.[23] Salient clinical features of photoaging include fine and coarse wrinkles, dyspigmentation, actinic keratoses, telangiectasias, and loss of elasticity. Sun-induced cutaneous changes vary among individuals, depending on age, gender, geographic location, and skin type, reflecting intrinsic differences in vulnerability and repair capacity.[24] Male gender has been shown a risk factor for photoaging for behavioral and biological reasons. Although photodamage can be partially prevented and reversed with proper sun protection (sunscreens and protective clothing), men tend not comply to these measures. One study found that 41% of men never apply sunscreen.[25] A recent multicenter cross-sectional study using a population-based survey of 416 individuals over the age of 18 years showed that men were more than twice less likely to put on sunscreen every day compared with men.[26] The reduced innate antioxidant capacity of men's skin translates into increased susceptibility to the catastrophic consequences of ROS accumulation. Beyond the undesirable cosmetic effects, the increased incidence in men of skin cancer,[27] both benign and malignant, stand testament to the detrimental impact of photoaging.[28]

Tobacco use is another lifestyle factor that accelerates the aging process, and men hold the lead when it comes to smoking. In 2012, the worldwide prevalence of smoking in men was 31.1% and 10.6% in women, while, according to the latest statistics, the age-standardized prevalence of daily smoking was 25% for men and 5% for women.[24] Smoking has detrimental effects to many organs because it contains several carcinogenic compounds and is a known cause of several diseases, such as cancer, asthma, and so forth. Smoking also has profound effects on the skin and aggravates cutaneous aging. A clinical study found cigarette smoking an independent risk

factor for the development of accelerated facial wrinkling and that the risk was dose dependent to smoking exposure.[25] Although the mechanism via which smoking affects the skin is not completely understood, factors include vasoconstriction, increased oxidative damage, and altered connective tissue metabolism.[29] Peripheral blood flow decreases by 30% to 40% within minutes after smoke inhalation, compromising tissue oxygenation, whereas inhibition of fibroblast activity and up-regulation of matrix metalloproteinase leads to decreased collagen synthesis and accumulation of ROS. Smoking is strongly associated with the development of facial elastosis and telangiectasias in men.[30] Elastotic skin is less elastic, dryer, darker, and more erythematous than normal skin.[31]

SUMMARY

The increased demand of aesthetic treatments for the face and body by men of all ages and ethnicities merits a complete and thorough understanding of male anatomy and the distinct pathophysiology of male aging for practicing dermatologists to provide the best patient consultation and treatment strategies. Unfortunately, despite the fact that the male patient population has been increasing for some years now, there is still paucity of information and clinical studies that analyze aesthetic treatments, technical details, and clinical results specifically for men. Popular cosmetic interventions particularly on the aged male face, such as neurotoxins and fillers, need to be carefully customized to avoid feminizing or leading to distorted results. Moreover, a cosmetic consultation needs to include patient education so male patients can embrace new habits that maintain treatment results and do not accelerate the aging process, such as use of sunscreens, cessation of smoking, and so forth. The medical community together with the male patients can bridge the existing gap pertinent to the advantage women have in terms of clinician experience to treat them, and all patients can enjoy equality in the pursuit of beauty.

REFERENCES

1. Com-, A.S.f.A.P.S.S. and p.c. 1997–2014. Available at: https://www.surgery.org/media/statistics. Accessed May 2, 2016.
2. Bokov A, Chaudhuri A, Richardson A. The role of oxidative damage and stress in aging. Mech Ageing Dev 2004;125(10–11):811–26.
3. Harman SM, Metter EJ, Tobin JD, et al. Longitudinal effects of aging on serum total and free testosterone

levels in healthy men. Baltimore longitudinal study of aging. J Clin Endocrinol Metab 2001;86(2):724–31.

4. Borras C, Gambini J, Gómez-Cabrera MC, et al. 17beta-oestradiol up-regulates longevity-related, antioxidant enzyme expression via the ERK1 and ERK2[MAPK]/NFkappaB cascade. Aging Cell 2005;4(3):113–8.

5. Ide T, Tsutsui H, Ohashi N, et al. Greater oxidative stress in healthy young men compared with premenopausal women. Arterioscler Thromb Vasc Biol 2002;22(3):438–42.

6. Viña J, Borrás C, Gambini J, et al. Why females live longer than males: control of longevity by sex hormones. Sci Aging Knowledge Environ 2005; 2005(23):pe17.

7. Fleg JL, Strait J. Accelerated longitudinal decline of aerobic capacity in healthy older adults. Circulation 2005;112(5):674–82.

8. Bulpitt CJ, Markowe HL, Shipley MJ. Why do some people look older than they should? Postgrad Med J 2001;77(911):578–81.

9. Giacomoni PU, Mammone T, Teri M. Gender-linked differences in human skin. J Dermatol Sci 2009; 55(3):144–9.

10. Wysong A, Kim D, Joseph T, et al. Quantifying soft tissue loss in the aging male face using magnetic resonance imaging. Dermatol Surg 2014;40(7): 786–93.

11. Montagna W, Carlisle K. Structural changes in ageing skin. Br J Dermatol 1990;122(Suppl 35): 61–70.

12. Yaar M, Gilchrest BA. Skin aging: postulated mechanisms and consequent changes in structure and function. Clin Geriatr Med 2001;17(4):617–30, v.

13. McCullough JL, Kelly KM. Prevention and treatment of skin aging. Ann N Y Acad Sci 2006;1067:323–31.

14. Deschenes MR. Effects of aging on muscle fibre type and size. Sports Med 2004;34(12):809–24.

15. Janssen I, Heymsfield SB, Wang ZM, et al. Skeletal muscle mass and distribution in 468 men and women aged 18-88 yr. J Appl Physiol (1985) 2000; 89(1):81–8.

16. Weeden JC, Trotman CA, Faraway JJ. Three dimensional analysis of facial movement in normal adults: influence of sex and facial shape. Angle Orthod 2001;71(2):132–40.

17. Shearer BM, Sholts SB, Garvin HM, et al. Sexual dimorphism in human browridge volume measured from 3D models of dry crania: a new digital morphometrics approach. Forensic Sci Int 2012;222(1–3): 400.e1-5.

18. Garvin HM, Ruff CB. Sexual dimorphism in skeletal browridge and chin morphologies determined using a new quantitative method. Am J Phys Anthropol 2012;147(4):661–70.

19. Zamboni M, Rossi AP, Fantin F, et al. Adipose tissue, diet and aging. Mech Ageing Dev 2014;136-137: 129–37.

20. Sjostrom L, Smith U, Krotkiewski M, et al. Cellularity in different regions of adipose tissue in young men and women. Metabolism 1972;21(12):1143–53.

21. Wysong A, Kim D, Joseph T, et al. Quantifying soft tissue loss in facial aging: a study in women using magnetic resonance imaging. Dermatol Surg 2013; 39(12):1895–902.

22. Ezure T, Yagi E, Kunizawa N, et al. Comparison of sagging at the cheek and lower eyelid between male and female faces. Skin Res Technol 2011; 17(4):510–5.

23. Yaar M, Gilchrest BA. Photoageing: mechanism, prevention and therapy. Br J Dermatol 2007; 157(5):874–87.

24. Malvy J, Guinot C, Preziosi P, et al. Epidemiologic determinants of skin photoaging: baseline data of the SU.VI.MAX. cohort. J Am Acad Dermatol 2000; 42(1 Pt 1):47–55.

25. Thieden E, Philipsen PA, Sandby-Møller J, et al. Sunscreen use related to UV exposure, age, sex, and occupation based on personal dosimeter readings and sun-exposure behavior diaries. Arch Dermatol 2005;141(8):967–73.

26. Lee A, Dixit S, Brown P, et al. The influence of age and gender in knowledge, behaviors and attitudes towards sun protection: a cross-sectional survey of Australian outpatient clinic attendees. Am J Clin Dermatol 2015;16(1):47–54.

27. Damian DL, Patterson CR, Stapelberg M, et al. UV radiation-induced immunosuppression is greater in men and prevented by topical nicotinamide. J Invest Dermatol 2008;128(2):447–54.

28. Dal H, Boldemann C, Lindelof B. Trends during a half century in relative squamous cell carcinoma distribution by body site in the Swedish population: support for accumulated sun exposure as the main risk factor. J Dermatol 2008;35(2):55–62.

29. Gill JF, Yu SS, Neuhaus IM. Tobacco smoking and dermatologic surgery. J Am Acad Dermatol 2013; 68(1):167–72.

30. Daling JR, Sherman KJ, Hislop TG, et al. Cigarette smoking and the risk of anogenital cancer. Am J Epidemiol 1992;135(2):180–9.

31. Model D. Smoker's face: an underrated clinical sign? Br Med J (Clin Res Ed) 1985;291(6511):1760–2.

Cosmetic Concerns Among Men

Marc Zachary Handler, MD[a,b,c],*, David J. Goldberg, MD, JD[a,b,d,e,f]

KEYWORDS

• Hair transplant • Submental fullness • Sexual dimorphism • Photo aging • Neuromodulators

KEY POINTS

• Men make up 10% of all cosmetic procedures.
• Men are concerned about looking feminized.
• Hair transplant and liposuction are the most common surgical procedures.
• Neuromodulators are the most common noninvasive cosmetic procedures.

The appearance of aging results from both internal factors, such as genetic predisposition, hormones, and free radicals, as well as external environmental factors, such as solar exposure. UV radiation is responsible for up to 90% of skin aging.[1] Commencing at age 30 years, men have an average reduction of testosterone of 1% per year.[1] A reduction in testosterone is correlated with a decreased thickness of male skin.[2] The combination of genetic, hormonal, and extrinsic factors lead to a loosening of elastic fibers and collagen, producing wrinkles and skin laxity.[1] Men also care about the presence of scalp hair. With regards to hair loss, a large concern among men, males differ from females in that testosterone and dihydrotestosterone play a role in androgenetic hair loss.[3]

A 2007 survey of men regarding their perception of cosmetic procedures revealed that 40% were interested in undergoing a cosmetic procedure.[4] For many men, an initial consultation, without anticipation of performing a specific procedure, is best performed to discuss their specific concerns. This is because men may be less familiar with cosmetic procedures and ask the physician

for help with a specific concerning area or simply request a global reduction in visual signs of aging.[5] When asked why men are reluctant to undergo cosmetic procedures, a common reason for hesitation was a fear of appearing feminized.[6] Men are acutely aware of the sexual dimorphism of facial features and wish to maintain or enhance traditionally masculine ones. An example is the different craniofacial shape between men and women.[7] As men develop confidence that physicians are able to maintain a masculine appearance, the number of men seeking cosmetic treatments will continue to increase. Despite the gap between women and men undergoing cosmetic procedures, as of 2015, men were consumers of close to 10% of all cosmetic treatments[6,8] (Fig. 1). This equates to a 325% increase in cosmetic procedures received by men since 1997.[9] There is an increased trend of nonsurgical interventions and decreased trend of surgical interventions. For those men undergoing surgical cosmetic procedures, the American Academy of Facial Plastic and Reconstructive Surgery reports the most frequent procedure performed

Disclosure Statement: The authors have nothing they wish to disclose.
[a] Skin Laser & Surgery Specialists, 115 E 57th Street, Suite 400, New York, NY 10022, USA; [b] Skin Laser & Surgery Specialists, 20 Prospect Avenue, Suite 702, Hackensack, NJ 07601, USA; [c] Dermatology, Rutgers New Jersey Medical School, 185 S Orange Avenue, Newark, NJ 07103, USA; [d] Dermatology, Icahn School of Medicine at Mt. Sinai, 5 E 98th Street, New York, NY 10029, USA; [e] Dermatology, Rutgers New Jersey Medical School, 185 South Orange Avenue, Medical Science Building H-576, Newark, NJ 07103-2757, USA; [f] Law, Fordham University School of Law, 150 W 62nd Street, New York, NY 10023, USA
* Corresponding author. Skin Laser & Surgery Specialists, 20 Prospect Avenue, Suite 702, Hackensack, NJ 07601.
E-mail address: drhandler@skinandlasers.com

Dermatol Clin 36 (2018) 5–10
https://doi.org/10.1016/j.det.2017.09.001
0733-8635/18/© 2017 Elsevier Inc. All rights reserved.

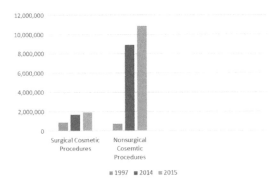

Fig. 1. Cosmetic procedures for both men and women.

is hair transplant, followed by rhinoplasty, blepharoplasty, scar revision, and facelift (**Box 1**).[10] Dermatologists report that the most frequent noninvasive cosmetic procedure is neuromodulator injections.[11] Jagdeo and colleagues[12] asked 600 men, primarily Caucasian, aged 30 to 65 years, what cosmetic concerns they had. Among that group, facial wrinkles were of concern to 48%; hair loss was a concern to 40%, and appearance of bags under the eyes was a concern to 44%. Dark under eye circles concerned 34%; sagging facial skin was a concern for 29%, and submental fat was a concern for 28%. Back hair was a concern among 20% (**Box 2**).[12] Pigmentation irregularities, such as lentigines and actinic damage were of concern to 30% to 34% of surveyed patients, respectively.[12] Ross and colleagues[13] reported that in San Diego pigmentation irregularities were the most common presenting concerns for men (**Box 3**). Men wish to achieve results that minimize apparent age, but maintain a masculine facial anatomy, requiring techniques that differ from than those used to treat women.

Throughout history, hair has been an important focus of social acceptability. The Romans learned to dye their hair, and the Egyptians wore wigs over close cut hair styles.[14] The terms big wig and bad hair day are examples that demonstrate the value

of hair in today's society. Scalp hair is a sign of youth, while back hair is not universally considered attractive; body hair removal represents 11.4% of male cosmetic treatments.

DHT, an androgen that results from conversion of testosterone by 5-α-reductase in hair follicles, results in male androgenetic hair loss by reduction of the hair's growth phase.[15] Male hair loss most often results from genetics and aging, with most men demonstrating some degree of androgenetic hair loss by 50 years of age.[3,16] A reduction in scalp hair may negatively impact a man's self-esteem.[3,16] Sixty-six percent of men with androgenetic alopecia wish they had more hair.[16] Sixty-two percent of men reported being teased about hair loss.[16,17] These rates of male dissatisfaction with hair loss have been found the United

---

Box 2
Top 10 cosmetic issue men are most concerned about

1. Facial wrinkles
2. Under eye bags
3. Hair loss
4. Facial sun damage
5. Dark under eye circles
6. Brown age spots
7. Sagging facial skin
8. Submental fullness
9. Brow ptosis
10. Back hair

From Jagdeo J, Keaney T, Narurkar V, et al. Facial treatment preferences among aesthetically oriented men. Dermatol Surg 2016;42(10):1160; with permission.

Box 1
Top 5 most common facial cosmetic surgeries in men

1. Hair transplant
2. Rhinoplasty
3. Blepharoplasty
4. Scar revision
5. Facelift

From Holcomb JD, Gentile RD. Aesthetic facial surgery of male patients: demographics and market trends. Facial Plast Surg 2005;21(4):225; with permission.

Box 3
10 most common presenting cosmetic concerns for men

1. Poikiloderma
2. Acne scars
3. Telangiectasia
4. Static pigmentation–lentigines
5. Dynamic pigmentation (melisma)
6. Seborrheic keratosis
7. Sebaceous hyperplasia
8. Shaving bumps and folliculitis
9. Wrinkles
10. Jowls

States and in Europe.[18] Men who are not in romantic relationships are at greater psychological risk, as they may feel their chances for acquiring a mate are reduced. Balding men may attempt to compensate for hair loss through changes to their physical appearance. Twenty-percent of men with hair loss grow facial hair, and 39% increase their amount of excerise.[16,17] Reducing the visible hair loss is an additional factor practiced among balding men, with 65% changing their hair style,[16] and 32% wearing a hat.[17] Although self-treatments, such as minoxidil, are available, men who feel the treatment is inadequate may have increased concern about hair loss.[17] Among facial plastic surgeons, male hair transplant remains the number one surgical cosmetic procedure performed.[10]

The sexual dimorphism of facial anatomy is of importance to men seeking cosmetic treatments. Unlike women who have prominent upper facial features, with a tapering heart shape, men have a square, angled jaw with equally proportioned features of the upper and lower face.[19] This impacts what men are interested in receiving, with regards to cosmetic filler. Men prefer to maintain a masculine appearance when receiving injectable filler treatments to restore facial volume loss. They wish to keep the youthful appearance at the malar eminence but want less cheek projection than would be seen in a woman.[20] This natural reduction in malar projection results from men having an average of 3 mm less subcutaneous malar fat than women.[21] The cheek is a common filler location in men, but too large an amount placed medial or lateral will feminize the face.[22] Men also are concerned about under eye festooning and deep tear troughs. Compared with women, men develop a tear trough deformity at a later age. This may explain why the men feel the presence of such a feature is unattractive, as it associated with frality.[19] The continued male concern with malar reduction and periorbital aging is the reason men are currently 7.4% of all patients receiving hyaluronic acid filler.[9] As opposed to women, lip filler is not a commonly requested procedure among men, as a large upper lip may be viewed as feminine.[22] As a whole, men have naturally thinner upper lips than women.[23] With age, lips thin in both sexes, but volume augmentation in men is considered taboo.[23] If requested to use filler in a man's lips, clear communication and expertise are a necessity.[23] Among injectables, hyaluronic acid is less commonly requested a procedure than neurotoxins.

In the Merchant of Venice, Shakespeare writes "with mirth and laughter let old wrinkles come." This may have been self-assuring in the sixteenth century, but in the twenty-first century, adult life expectancy is no longer only 60 years, and packaged botulinum neurotoxin type A is available.[24] In men, the forehead is most susceptible to wrinkles, the hallmark of photo aging.[25] The depth of wrinkles results from their thicker skin and facial musculature, as well as propensity to not adopt sun-protective behaviors.[6,26] Additionally, men have greater muscle mass and muscle movement of the face than women. This explains why men develop deep facial furrows.[27] When surveyed on the issue, 60% of men were concerned about the appearance of their glabellar lines.[12] Consequently, the male increased muscle mass of the glabella area requires an increased dosage of botulinum toxin, up to 5 times more, than is needed to treat the same area in women.[28] Physicians who treat men with neurotoxins must recognize that standard doses used in women may not be sufficient to produce a result in men's brows, and be conscious that insufficient dosing is not a result of product ineffectiveness.[29] Although interest in neurotoxins is increasing among millennial men,[30] it is men in their sixth decade who are peaking in their careers and aware that they have aged and developed wrinkles. They also have reached a point of confidence with their position in life, but are afraid of looking aged. Among this group there is a fine balance that must be struck between maintaining a few wrinkles, in order to inspire trust, and having too many, which is perceived as brittle.[31] When men between the ages of 55 and 59 years were asked the reason for their interest wrinkle reduction, 51% stated they wished to look more youthful, and 16% stated that they felt it would help them maintain a competitive edge in the workforce.[12] The area where wrinkling is most concerning to men is the forehead.[12] Neurotoxin use in the corrugators and glabella without treatment of the frontalis will produce an elevated brow, a feminine feature. Men prefer a horizontal brow, requiring treatment of the frontalis muscle, if the glabella area is treated.[32] Crow's feet and tear troughs are also of concern to men. This may result from the importance that eyes play in society, but it is also known that men develop more severe facial rhytids than women.[6,33] This has not directly correlated to having severe rhytids treated, as men currently represent only 10.3% of patients receiving neurotoxin.[9] But that percentage has increased by greater than 80% over the prior 6 years.[22] The number of men receiving neurotoxin for cosmetic reasons is expected to rise as there is an increase in social acceptability of cosmetic procedures among men and an increased understanding of the minimal post-treatment recovery time.[11]

Men wish to minimize love handles and acquire a V-shaped torso, where the body's greatest width is the shoulders, and narrowest the waist. The contoured physique is as old as antiquity, highlighted by the famous Belvedere Torso, which dates to first century BC, and the inspiration for Michelangelo's Adam, which he painted on the Sistine Chapel.[34] In order to achieve this, body contouring remains a large cosmetic request among men. A Turkish survey found that 53% of men considered surgical body contouring, such as liposuction, for improvement of physique.[35] The most common surgical cosmetic procedure for men as of 2015 was liposuction of the abdomen.[9] The fourth was surgical reduction of gynecomastia (**Box 4**).[36,37] Among liposuction cases performed between both sexes, 13% are and 50 years.[9] It is not only the abdomen that men are concerned about. Since 1997, male surgical breast reduction has increased by 173%, and increased 26% since 2014.[9] Male breast reduction procedures peak in the 19- to 34-year-old demographic.[9] Gynecomastia, an increase in glandular tissue and pseudogynecomastia, resulting from excess subareolar fat, exists in 40% and 64% of men, respectively.[38] Although surgical treatment may target both true gynecomastia and pseudogynecomastia, noninvasive treatments, such as cryolipolysis, have been successfully utilized to decrease subareolar fat.[38] With social pressure to maintain a trim figure and an increased number of noninvasive fat reduction systems, including cryolipolysis, radiofrequency, high-intensity focused ultrasound, and low-level laser therapy, it should be no surprise that men represent 16.7% of all nonsurgical fat reduction procedures.[9] For men who seek even greater weight loss, bariatric surgery is an option. As of 2011, 19.3% of all patients undergoing bariatric surgery were men.[39] After substantial weight loss, such as from bariatric surgery, there is an interest in lower body lifting to remove redundant tissue. Among those undergoing surgical lower body lifts, men represented 13.0% of cases.[9]

Since the golden age of filmmaking, actors with strong chins, such as Kirk Douglas and Cary Grant, have been viewed as sex symbols. This may help explain why the lower face is an area about which men are particularly concerned.[40] Among men, 70% are concerned about the appearance of submental fullness. From 2014 to 2015, there was a 58% increase in nonsurgical skin tightening, including reduction of jowls and submental fat as well as nonsurgical body contouring.[9] It should be no surprise that men will continue to seek improvement in this area as long as a chiseled jaw, epitomized by superheroes such as Superman, remains the masculine ideal.

The reason for an increase in men wanting and willing to seek cosmetic treatments is unclear.[41] Studies have found that there is an association between increased income and increased attractiveness. It has also been hypothesized that, similar to women, there is an increased media pressure on men to maintain a certain physical appearance.[41] Television and magazines celebrate a youthful appearance and reject the elderly. Whatever the reason, as with women, men are looking to compete both socially and financially by augmenting their appearance.[10] Currently the primary male consumer of cosmetic procedures is aged 40 to 59 years, with discretionary income.[10] This average age is anticipated to widen as the baby boomer generation enters their 60s and 70s.[5] Male concerns about cosmetic interventions include safety (46%), cost (42%), and fear of appearing unnatural (41%) (**Box 5**).[12] Hair loss topped the list of male cosmetic concerns.[12] This was followed by concern of the appearance of submental fullness and deep tear troughs.[12] Crow's feet and forehead rhytids were concerning to 15% and 18% of men, respectively.[12] Unlike women, men were not distressed about the appearance of their eyelashes, lips, or perioral rhytids.[12] Although there is a slow increase in

---

Box 4
Top 5 most common cosmetic surgeries for men per the American Society for Aesthetic Plastic Surgery

1. Liposuction
2. Rhinoplasty
3. Blepharoplasty
4. Male breast reduction
5. Facelift

Box 5
Why men may avoid injectables

1. Feel they do not yet need injectables
2. Side effect risk
3. Safety concern about injecting a foreign substance
4. Cost
5. Concern results will look unnatural

From Jagdeo J, Keaney T, Narurkar V, et al. Facial treatment preferences among aesthetically oriented men. Dermatol Surg 2016;42(10):1162; with permission.

adoption of cosmetic procedures among men, more education may be needed to reduce the anxiety regarding safety and unnatural or masculine appearance. Physicians should be ready to assist men in determining their concerns. As men often seek treatment at the behest of a loved one, they may be unable to articulate their concerns clearly.[13]

REFERENCES

1. Keaney TC. Aging in the male face: intrinsic and extrinsic factors. Dermatol Surg 2016;42(7): 797–803.
2. Panyakhamlerd K, Chotnopparatpattara P, Taechakraichana N, et al. Skin thickness in different menopausal status. J Med Assoc Thai 1999;82(4): 352–6.
3. Park S, Erdogan S, Hwang D, et al. Bee venom promotes hair growth in association with inhibiting 5alpha-reductase expression. Biol Pharm Bull 2016;39(6):1060–8.
4. Frederick DA, Lever J, Peplau LA. Interest in cosmetic surgery and body image: views of men and women across the lifespan. Plast Reconstr Surg 2007;120(5):1407–15.
5. Wieczorek IT, Hibler BP, Rossi AM. Injectable cosmetic procedures for the male patient. J Drugs Dermatol 2015;14(9):1043–51.
6. Keaney T. Male aesthetics. Skin Therapy Lett 2015; 20(2):5–7.
7. Goldstein SM, Katowitz JA. The male eyebrow: a topographic anatomic analysis. Ophthal Plast Reconstr Surg 2005;21(4):285–91.
8. ASDS survey: half of consumers considering cosmetic procedure. 2015. Available at: https://www.asds.net/_Media.aspx?id=8963. Accessed December 30, 2016.
9. Cosmetic surgery National Data Bank statistics. Aesthet Surg J 2016;36(Suppl 1):1–29.
10. Holcomb JD, Gentile RD. Aesthetic facial surgery of male patients: demographics and market trends. Facial Plast Surg 2005;21(4):223–31.
11. Keaney TC, Alster TS. Botulinum toxin in men: review of relevant anatomy and clinical trial data. Dermatol Surg 2013;39(10):1434–43.
12. Jagdeo J, Keaney T, Narurkar V, et al. Facial treatment preferences among aesthetically oriented men. Dermatol Surg 2016;42(10):1155–63.
13. Ross EV. Nonablative laser rejuvenation in men. Dermatol Ther 2007;20(6):414–29.
14. Haas N, Toppe F, Henz BM. Hairstyles in the arts of Greek and Roman antiquity. J Investig Dermatol Symp Proc 2005;10(3):298–300.
15. Itami S, Kurata S, Takayasu S. 5 alpha-reductase activity in cultured human dermal papilla cells from beard compared with reticular dermal fibroblasts. J Invest Dermatol 1990;94(1):150–2.
16. Cash TF. The psychological effects of androgenetic alopecia in men. J Am Acad Dermatol 1992;26(6): 926–31.
17. Cash TF. The psychology of hair loss and its implications for patient care. Clin Dermatol 2001;19(2): 161–6.
18. Budd D, Himmelberger D, Rhodes T, et al. The effects of hair loss in European men: a survey in four countries. Eur J Dermatol 2000;10(2):122–7.
19. de Maio M. Ethnic and gender considerations in the use of facial injectables: male patients. Plast Reconstr Surg 2015;136(5 Suppl):40S–3S.
20. Why men have different facial filler needs. Elevate 2012.
21. Codinha S. Facial soft tissue thicknesses for the Portuguese adult population. Forensic Sci Int 2009; 184(1–3):80.e1-7.
22. Farhadian JA, Bloom BS, Brauer JA. Male aesthetics: a review of facial anatomy and pertinent clinical implications. J Drugs Dermatol 2015;14(9): 1029–34.
23. Chatham DR. Special considerations for the male patient: things I wish I knew when I started practice. Facial Plast Surg 2005;21(4):232–9.
24. Plantation P. Raising children in the early 17th century: demographics. edmaterials_demographics. Available at: https://www.plimoth.org/sites/default/files/media/pdf/edmaterials_demographics.pdf. Accessed December 31, 2016.
25. Luebberding S, Krueger N, Kerscher M. Quantification of age-related facial wrinkles in men and women using a three-dimensional fringe projection method and validated assessment scales. Dermatol Surg 2014;40(1):22–32.
26. Sattler U, Thellier S, Sibaud V, et al. Factors associated with sun protection compliance: results from a nationwide cross-sectional evaluation of 2215 patients from a dermatological consultation. Br J Dermatol 2014;170(6):1327–35.
27. Weeden JC, Trotman CA, Faraway JJ. Three dimensional analysis of facial movement in normal adults: influence of sex and facial shape. Angle Orthod 2001;71(2):132–40.
28. Brandt F, Swanson N, Baumann L, et al. Randomized, placebo-controlled study of a new botulinum toxin type a for treatment of glabellar lines: efficacy and safety. Dermatol Surg 2009;35(12):1893–901.
29. Jones D. Gentlemen, relax: commentary on botulinum toxin in men: a review of relevant anatomy and clinical trial data. Dermatol Surg 2013;39(10): 1444–5.
30. Lalani A. Millennials using Botox to stay young looking, plastic surgeons say. Toronto Journal Star 2016. Life.
31. Harper J. 'Dramatic' increase: plastic surgery for men up by 43 percent as they compete in the job market. The Washington Times 2015. National.

32. Bloom JD, Green JB, Bowe W, et al. Cosmetic use of abobotulinumtoxin A in men: considerations regarding anatomical differences and product characteristics. J Drugs Dermatol 2016;15(9):1056–62.

33. Tsukahara K, Hotta M, Osanai O, et al. Gender-dependent differences in degree of facial wrinkles. Skin Res Technol 2013;19(1):e65–71.

34. Clark N. Vatican to loan famed Belvedere Torso to British museum. 2015. Available at: http://www.independent.co.uk/arts-entertainment/art/news/vatican-to-loan-famed-belvedere-torso-to-british-museum-9965865.html. Accessed December 31, 2016.

35. Ozel B, Sezgin B, Guney K, et al. A social evaluation of perception on body contouring surgery by Turkish male aesthetic surgery patients. Aesthetic Plast Surg 2015;39(1):124–8.

36. Surgery TASfAaP. Cosmetic surgery National Data Bank statistics 2015. 2015. Available at: http://www.surgery.org/sites/default/files/ASAPS-Stats2015.pdf. Accessed December 14, 2016.

37. Singh B, Keaney T, Rossi AM. Male body contouring. J Drugs Dermatol 2015;14(9):1052–9.

38. Munavalli GS, Panchaprateep R. Cryolipolysis for targeted fat reduction and improved appearance of the enlarged male breast. Dermatol Surg 2015; 41(9):1043–51.

39. Young MT, Phelan MJ, Nguyen NT. A decade analysis of trends and outcomes of male vs female patients who underwent bariatric surgery. J Am Coll Surg 2016;222(3):226–31.

40. Remnick D. Donald Trump personally blasts the press. The New Yorker 2016.

41. Leitermann M, Hoffmann K, Kasten E. What's preventing us to get more attraction: the fear of aesthetic surgery. World J Plast Surg 2016;5(3): 226–35.

Cosmetic Concerns Among Ethnic Men

 CrossMark

Michelle Henry, MD

KEYWORDS

• Ethnic • Men • Skin • Rejuvenation

KEY POINTS

- Cultural, pathophysiologic, and anatomic differences in ethnic skin require different treatment approaches than those offered to fair skinned patients.
- Hyperpigmentation and scarring are the most prevalent adverse effects that limit the use of certain treatment modalities such as laser/light therapies.
- Sun protection is imperative for prevention and maintenance of treatment results in ethnic men.

INTRODUCTION

The demand for cosmetic procedures is on the increase in the male population of all ethnic groups. According to the latest statistics from the American Society for Aesthetic Plastic Surgery, more than 1,000,000 cosmetic procedures (both invasive and minimally invasive) were performed in men in 2015, and 25% of the individuals undergoing treatments were men of color. Although no standard classification system exists for skin of color, it is common for physicians to use the Fitzpatrick skin types categories, originally developed to describe the response to UV light in phototherapy. Using the Fitzpatrick system, olive/beige tones are classified as type IV, brown skin as type V, and black skin as type VI. In the United States, people from Africa, the Caribbean, Asia, Pacific Islands, Latin America, Native Americans, Latino, Hispanics, Indians, and those of Middle Eastern origin are considered to have ethnic skin.

There is a the paucity of clinical data and studies specifically examining cosmetic concerns in ethnic men, given that this is a growing population with distinct needs regarding gender and skin physiology, it is important for dermatologists to be aware how to treat, counsel, and address the needs of this patient cohort. In fact, a survey conducted in dermatologists in Australia showed that 85% of participants were not confident in managing common cosmetic issues in skin of color, and more than 80% stated they would have liked more teaching in skin of color.[1]

The skin pathophysiology in ethnic individuals has biological differences when compared with fair skin that affect cosmetic treatment needs. Because of the increased melanin, patients with darker skin have inherent protection against extrinsic factors of aging such as damage from UV, and photoaging appears decades later compared with those with lighter skin tones. Photodamage is typically manifested as pigmentary aberrations (lentigines, macules, melasma) rather than rhytides. Moreover, facial aging in patients of color is due to volume loss from deeper muscular layers than dermal layers. Perioral and periorbital lines may not occur as early in patients of color, but there is a tendency toward mid and lower face aging, with manifestations including the formation of nasolabial folds and sagging of the jowl.[2,3] Skin of patients of color also have thicker more compact dermis and stratum corneum with more cornified layers.[4]

Hair structure is also different in patients of color patients. Black individuals have flat elliptical-shaped hair shafts with curved hair follicles, and

Disclosure: M. Henry has nothing to disclose.
Department of Dermatology, Weill Cornell Medicine, 1 Irving Place, Apartment G21B, 1305 York Avenue, New York, NY 10065, USA
E-mail address: michelle.HenryMD@gmail.com

derm.theclinics.com

fewer elastic fibers anchoring hair follicles to the dermis, whereas the Asian hair shaft is round with the largest cross-sectional area.[5,6]

Aside from the differences in skin pathophysiology and anatomy in patients of color, there are profound cultural differences that dictate cosmetic concerns, habits, and goals. Ethnic men have historically been hesitant to pursue cosmetic treatments because of fears of being viewed as rejecting their racial identity. As techniques have advanced, and physicians have developed a nuanced and culturally/gender-sensitive approach to beauty, ethnic men can now share cosmetic goals similar to their Caucasian counterpart men. Enhancing physical appearance and combating aging is a shared goal because it is tied to personal success in life.

ANTIAGING TREATMENTS FOR ETHNIC MEN

Restoring a youthful appearance is a common goal of ethnic men, and dermatologists can offer several treatment options either as monotherapy or in a combination approach. Energy-based devices such as those that harness energy from laser/lights and radiofrequency in combination with fillers/neurotoxins and topical cosmeceuticals can reduce the appearance of wrinkles, pore size, and laxity and replete any areas of volume loss.

Lasers

Nonablative fractional laser resurfacing can be considered among first-line therapy for the reduction of fine lines and wrinkling, textural abnormalities, and pore size in ethnic male patients, because it has an excellent safety profile and short downtime. Fractional photothermolysis creates microscopic columns of thermal injury that have a diameter ranging from 100 to 160 μm with a depth of penetration 300 to 700 μm. Because epidermal and follicular structures are spared and melanin is not at risk of targeted destruction, nonablative fractional laser resurfacing can be used successfully in patients with skin of color. Suitable candidates include those with mild/moderate photodamage acne scarring and striae. Caution should be taken in patients with melasma or keloid scars. An ideal treatment regimen has been shown to typically include a series of 4 to 6 treatments with low densities allowing for adequate recovery between sessions. Often pretreatment and posttreatment with hydroquinone-containing creams are useful to prevent hyperpigmentation.

In a retrospective review of 362 patients undergoing nonablative fractional laser treatments with either 1550-nm erbium or 1927-nm thulium fiber laser, postinflammatory hyperpigmentation occurred in only 1.1% of patients, whereas worsening of melasma was noted in 0.9% of cases.[7] Kono and colleagues[8] also demonstrated the safety and efficacy of nonablative fractional 1550 nm laser in patients of color, noting that patient satisfaction was higher when their skin is treated with high fluences than with high densities. Another study using the fractionated nonablative 1440-nm laser in 20 patients (skin types I-VI) showed that 6 treatments were generally required to achieve a significant reduction in pore size.[9]

Radiofrequency

Radiofrequency devices that emit thermal energy to the dermal layers of the skin can stimulate wound-healing mechanisms promoting collagen production and remodeling that ultimately leads to skin rejuvenation. Radiofrequency treatments are safe for all skin types because thermal energy is chromophore independent; thus epidermal melanin is not at risk of destruction. Early generations of radiofrequency devices such as the monopolar Thermage (Solta, Hayward, CA, USA) have been shown to be effective in improving periorbital and jowl laxity in patients of darker skin types.[10] More recently, new generations of technologies, such as that of fractional microneedle radiofrequency, have also been tested for skin rejuvenation in dark skinned patients. Subjects receiving 3 treatments of fractionated microneedle radiofrequency at 4-week intervals experienced clinical improvement in areas such as periorbital wrinkling and high patient satisfaction at the 6-month follow-up.[11]

Microfocused Ultrasound

Microfocused ultrasound technologies (MFU) deliver ultrasound energy to the reticular dermis, and by producing microcoagulation zones, stimulate denaturation, collagen remodeling, and skin rejuvenation without influencing the epidermal layer. Because the energy is not selectively absorbed by chromophores, MFU is safe for darker complexions that have excess laxity. A recent clinical study demonstrated the safety and efficacy of MFU for improving laxity of the skin of the face and neck in 52 adults with Fitzpatrick skin types III to VI. No adverse events were reported, and side effects including erythema self-resolved in the weeks following treatment.[12]

Toxins

Brow furrows, glabellar creases, and crow's feet resulting from hyperfunctional facial muscles manifests equally in men and women of all races.

Moreover, although men seek treatments with neurotoxins to appear more relaxed and youthful, there is also a need for conservative treatments and preservation of some movement to attain a natural appearance and avoid feminization. Prominent and full male eyebrows without a significant arch enhance masculinity. Thus, regardless of race, treatment with neurotoxins should preserve a lower position of the brows and a flatter arch. Botulinum toxin-A is the most common neurotoxin used for the relaxation of glabellar frown lines and off-label for relaxation of the upper and lower hyperkinetic muscles in patients of color.[13,14] Treatments with toxins should precede at least 2 weeks before treatments with fillers because injections with botulinum toxin can reduce the amount of fillers needed to correct creases and folds. A common goal specific to Asians is the desire to achieve a more open eyelid, and clinically this can be achieved by injecting 1 to 2 units of botulinum toxin-A into the mid lower lid that preserves the shape of the Asian but opens the eye slightly.[15]

Fillers

As mentioned earlier, although people of darker skin have thicker dermis and less perioral/periorbital rhytides, they do experience age-related muscle and volume loss, thus often seek treatments for volume repletion. Because of the reduced rate of collagen degradation in ethnic skin and the collagen-stimulating properties of new generation fillers, fewer treatments are usually necessary to achieve desired volume restoration. The most common fillers used in men include calcium hydroxylapatite (Radiesse; Merz Aesthetics, Raleigh, NC, USA), poly-L-lactic acid (Galderma, Fort Worth, TX, USA), and hyaluronic acid (Juvederm; Allergan, Parsippany-Troy Hills, NJ, USA) (**Fig. 1**). When injecting fillers in skin of color, one of the most important technical considerations is minimizing the use of multiple puncture techniques. In a clinical trial of 150 patients (skin types IV–VI), multiple puncture technique was associated with a 13% incidence of hyperpigmentation compared with lineal threading technique, whereby the incidence of hyperpigmentation was merely 2%. Adverse effects such as postinflammatory hyperpigmentation and ecchymosis can be reduced with slower injection rates.[16,17]

SKIN TONE AND PIGMENTATION DISORDERS

Treating uneven skin tone and disorders of pigmentation, including postinflammatory hyperpigmentation and melasma, are particularly concerning in men of color. The prevalence of melasma in men has been estimated to approximately 20%, and it is generally recognized to be more common in individuals with Fitzpatrick skin types IV–VI.[18] Treatment of melasma or pigmentary disorders is generally similar for both genders and includes modalities such as topical medications, chemical peels, lasers, and light treatment. When treating men, however, it is important to consider there is a tendency for men to invest in simple, quick therapeutic strategies and that they are less compliant to approaches that entail incorporating multistep therapies in their daily routine. As melasma and similar pigmentary disorders are generally recognized to be caused by melanocyte overactivation, sun avoidance and rigorous application of sunscreen containing sun protection factor 30 or greater are a must. Men need to be counseled and understand that photoprotection underscores all treatment modalities for disorders of pigmentation, and without photoprotection, minimal benefit will be seen with any other therapeutic option.

Topical agents that have been successfully used for melasma and hyperpigmentary disorders include hydroquinone, azelaic acid, topical corticosteroid, kojic acid, arbutin, licorice extract, ascorbic acid, soy, and chemical peeling (glycolic acid, salicylic acid, trichloroacetic acid, retinoic acid).[19] Cosmeceutical formulations can be beneficial in darker skin for issues of uneven color and hyperpigmentation, such as Lytera (SkinMedica) and Phloretin (SkinCeuticals), a topical vitamin C product that is particularly well suited for deeper skin tones. Positive results have also been noted with the nutraceutical *Polypodium Leucotomos*, an oral antioxidant that has been shown to inhibit melanogenesis and can be safety consumed by patients of all skin types as monotherapy or for synergy with topical/energy-based treatments. Tranexamic acid has also been proven efficacious in reducing pigmentary conditions like melasma.

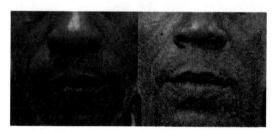

Fig. 1. A 50-year old man (skin type V) before (*left*) and 6 months after (*right*) Poly(methyl methacrylate) filler in the nasolabial folds. (*Courtesy of* Suneva Medical, San Diego, CA.)

Energy-based devices such as lasers and radio-frequency can also be beneficial for pigmentation disorders, but caution needs to be exercised when choosing the settings to prevent hypopigmentation, postinflammatory hyperpigmentation. Lasers with longer wavelengths such as the neodymium-doped yttrium aluminum garnet (Nd:YAG) 1064 nm laser can penetrate and target deep dermal melanin while sparing the epidermal normal melanin.[20,21] Picosecond lasers are also emerging as a new class of lasers that can be safe for dark skin because they destroy melanocytes via high-pressure photoacoustic effect, thus decreasing the thermal damage on surrounding structures[22] (Fig. 2).

Fractionated microneedle radiofrequency has also been recently reported to be effective in treating pigment issues in skin of color, either as a monotherapy or as a means of transdermal delivery of topicals. By creating zones of microablation in the deep dermis, these devices can improve texture, tone, and color in all skin types. Because melanin is not a target of the device, there is little to no risk of hyperpigmentation unless multiple pass treatments are used, thus inducing too high levels of ablation. A prospective randomized study comparing tranexamic acid microinjections to microneedling followed by topical tranexamic acid application in 60 patients (Fitzpatrick skin type IV–V) with moderate to severe melasma showed that the combination of microneedling with tranexamic acid was superior in improving the Melasma Area Severity Index score with no adverse effects reported.[23]

ACNE AND OTHER SCARRING

One of the most frequent dermatologic disorders observed in ethnic patients is acne, and in black patients, this condition is often accompanied by postinflammatory hyperpigmentation and scarring.[24,25] Moreover, likely because of increased fibroblast in the dermis, ethnic skin is more prone to hypertrophic scarring following injury, and keloid scar formation is reported to be 5 to 15 times higher in African Americans compared with the white population.[26,27] Treatment modalities for acne scars are similar for both men and women of darker skin types

and include chemical peels, microneedling, energy-based devices, and fillers. A study in 50 patients (skin types III–VI) showed that after 3 monthly microneedling sessions there was a statistically significant improvement of acne scars with no adverse effects reported.[28] Nonablative fractional lasers such as the 1440-nm Nd:YAG, 1550-nm Er:YAG laser, and 1927-nm thulium fiber laser can treat acne scars and rejuvenate the skin, but the results have been proven moderate for ethnic skin because of the conservative settings used to prevent pigmentation-related adverse effects.[29] According to the investigators' experience, one of the most successful strategies to reduce the appearance of scarring is the combination of fractionated microneedle radiofrequency with a permanent filler such as Bellafill (Suneva, Santa Barbara, CA, USA)[30,31] (Fig. 3). Microneedle radiofrequency can treat acne scarring through stimulating dermal remodeling and production of dermal components with minimal risk of dyspigmentation in patients with skin of color, whereas the US Food and Drug Administration–approved for acne scar filler Bellafill can seal areas of excess grooving and ridging.

HAIR DISORDERS

The differences in some ethnic men's hair structure paired with grooming habits have implications on the development of hair disorders, including pseudofolliculitis barbae and acne keloidalis nuchae. This is more commonly seen in men of African descent.

Pseudofolliculitis Barbae

This condition is a chronic noninfectious inflammatory condition prevalent in ethnic men. Clinical features include follicular and/or perifollicular

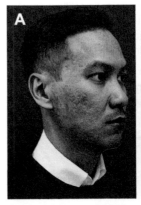
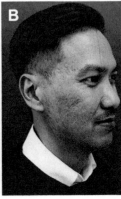

Fig. 3. A 30-year old (skin type IV) before (*A left*) and 6 months after (*B right*) 4 Tx with fractional microneedle radiofrequency. (*Courtesy of* Sadick Dermatology, New York.)

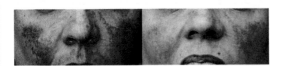

Fig. 2. A 44-year old man (skin type IV) before (*left*) and 12 months after (*right*) 2 treatment with 1064-nm picosecond laser. (*Courtesy of* Cutera Medical, Brisbane, CA.)

papules in the neck, chin, and sometimes the cheek area. Symptoms of pseudofolliculitis barbae include pain during or after shaving, itching, stinging, and diffuse pain on the skin. Although this condition was attributed to shaving habits, it is increasingly recognized to have a genetic basis. Simple changes in shaving routine have proven to decrease flaring of the condition, including use of a single blade razor, premoisturizing of shaving area, and hydration after shaving. In more severe cases where therapeutic intervention is necessary, various strategies have been successfully used, such as laser hair removal. The safest lasers for treating ethnic skin with pseudofolliculitis barbae is the long-pulse 1064-nm Nd:YAG laser, used with conservative settings (lower fluences and longer pulse durations) (**Fig. 4**). A study in 22 men (skin types IV–VI) with pseudofolliculitis barbae refractory to conservative therapy receiving 5 weekly treatments using 1064-nm Nd:YAG laser (12 J/cm^2, 20 ms, 10-mm spot size) demonstrated that 83% of patients had global improvement in the markers evaluated (dyspigmentation, papule count, cobblestoning) with no adverse effects.[32]

Acne Keloidalis Nuchae

This chronic condition is characterized by papules, pustules, and sometimes tumorous masses in the posterior region of the scalp.

Treatment strategies include topical steroids, systemic agents (antibiotics, retinoids), surgery, and recently, laser/light devices. Treatment with 1064-nm Nd:YAG and the 810-nm diode lasers have been found useful in reducing lesion count and size in patients with this condition by destroying the hair follicles within the lesions and reducing the inflammation.[33] Aside from treatment, change in hair care practices such as the use of electric clippers to groom the hair short, often seen in men of African ancestry, might play a role in reducing flare-ups. Mechanical factors, such as the friction from electric clippers, can exacerbate the condition; thus physicians should advise to decrease the use of anything that would create friction and aggravate papules on the back of the scalp.

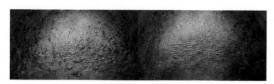

Fig. 4. 36-year old man (skin type VI) before (*left*) and 12 months after (*right*) 4 Tx with long pulsed 1064-nm Nd:YAG. (*Courtesy of* Cutera Medical, Brisbane, CA.)

SUMMARY

Ethnic men are an emerging patient cohort that seeks and invests in treatments to improve various aspects of their appearance, including but not limited to skin tone, texture, signs of aging, and hair disorders. Although these patients present inherent nuances and require that the treating physician is sensitized to their specific needs. There is now a plethora of treatment options available for these patients that are both effective and safe for their skin tone. Nevertheless, as the focus thus far when it comes to aesthetics has been dominated by the female gender, it is important that more clinical studies are tailored to evaluate specific technical protocols and regimes for ethnic men to provide better clinical care and meet to their needs more thoroughly.

REFERENCES

1. Rodrigues MA, Ross AL, Gilmore S, et al. Australian dermatologists' perspective on skin of colour: results of a national survey. Australas J Dermatol 2016. [Epub ahead of print].
2. Harris MO. The aging face in patients of color: minimally invasive surgical facial rejuvenation-a targeted approach. Dermatol Ther 2004;17:206–11.
3. Liew S, Wu WT, Chan HH, et al. Consensus on changing trends, attitudes, and concepts of asian beauty. Aesthetic Plast Surg 2016;40:193–201.
4. Taylor SC. Skin of color: biology, structure, function, and implications for dermatologic disease. J Am Acad Dermatol 2002;46:S41–62.
5. Montagna W, Carlisle K. The architecture of black and white facial skin. J Am Acad Dermatol 1991; 24:929–37.
6. Vernall DG. A study of the size and shape of cross sections of hair from four races of men. Am J Phys Anthropol 1961;19:345–50.
7. Lee SM, Kim MS, Kim YJ, et al. Adverse events of non-ablative fractional laser photothermolysis: a retrospective study of 856 treatments in 362 patients. J Dermatolog Treat 2014;25:304–7.
8. Kono T, Chan HH, Groff WF, et al. Prospective direct comparison study of fractional resurfacing using different fluences and densities for skin rejuvenation in Asians. Lasers Surg Med 2007;39:311–4.
9. Saedi N, Petrell K, Arndt K, et al. Evaluating facial pores and skin texture after low-energy nonablative fractional 1440-nm laser treatments. J Am Acad Dermatol 2013;68:113–8.
10. Kushikata N, Negishi K, Tezuka Y, et al. Non-ablative skin tightening with radiofrequency in Asian skin. Lasers Surg Med 2005;36:92–7.
11. Lee SJ, Kim JI, Yang YJ, et al. Treatment of periorbital wrinkles with a novel fractional radiofrequency

microneedle system in dark-skinned patients. Dermatol Surg 2015;41:615–22.

12. Harris MO, Sundaram HA. Safety of microfocused ultrasound with visualization in patients with Fitzpatrick skin phototypes III to VI. JAMA Facial Plast Surg 2015;17:355–7.

13. Burgess CM. Soft tissue augmentation in skin of color: market growth, available fillers, and successful techniques. J Drugs Dermatol 2007;6:51–5.

14. Carruthers JD, Carruthers A. Botulinum A exotoxin in clinical ophthalmology. Can J Ophthalmol 1996;31: 389–400.

15. Flynn TC, Carruthers JA, Carruthers JA. Botulinum-A toxin treatment of the lower eyelid improves infraorbital rhytides and widens the eye. Dermatol Surg 2001;27:703–8.

16. Hamilton TK, Burgess CM. Considerations for the use of injectable poly-L-lactic acid in people of color. J Drugs Dermatol 2010;9:451–6.

17. Taylor SC, Burgess CM, Callender VD. Safety of nonanimal stabilized hyaluronic acid dermal fillers in patients with skin of color: a randomized, evaluator-blinded comparative trial. Dermatol Surg 2009;35(Suppl 2):1653–60.

18. Vachiramon V, Suchonwanit P, Thadanipon K. Melasma in men. J Cosmet Dermatol 2012;11:151–7.

19. Gupta AK, Gover MD, Nouri K, et al. The treatment of melasma: a review of clinical trials. J Am Acad Dermatol 2006;55:1048–65.

20. Gokalp H, Akkaya AD, Oram Y. Long-term results in low-fluence 1064-nm Q-switched Nd:YAG laser for melasma: is it effective? J Cosmet Dermatol 2016; 15:420–6.

21. Yue B, Yang Q, Xu J, et al. Efficacy and safety of fractional Q-switched 1064-nm neodymium-doped yttrium aluminum garnet laser in the treatment of melasma in Chinese patients. Lasers Med Sci 2016;31:1657–63.

22. Ohshiro T, Ohshiro T, Sasaki K, et al. Picosecond pulse duration laser treatment for dermal melanocytosis in Asians: a retrospective review. Laser Ther 2016;25: 99–104.

23. Budamakuntla L, Loganathan E, Suresh DH, et al. A randomised, open-label, comparative study of tranexamic acid microinjections and tranexamic acid with microneedling in patients with melasma. J Cutan Aesthet Surg 2013;6:139–43.

24. Alexis AF. Acne vulgaris in skin of color: understanding nuances and optimizing treatment outcomes. J Drugs Dermatol 2014;13:s61–5.

25. Taylor SC, Cook-Bolden F, Rahman Z, et al. Acne vulgaris in skin of color. J Am Acad Dermatol 2002;46:S98–106.

26. Corcuff P, Lotte C, Rougier A, et al. Racial differences in corneocytes. A comparison between black, white and oriental skin. Acta Derm Venereol 1991; 71:146–8.

27. Leflore IC. Misconceptions regarding elective plastic surgery in the black patient. J Natl Med Assoc 1980;72:947–8.

28. Fabbrocini G, De Vita V, Monfrecola A, et al. Percutaneous collagen induction: an effective and safe treatment for post-acne scarring in different skin phototypes. J Dermatolog Treat 2014;25:147–52.

29. Britt CJ, Marcus B. Energy-based facial rejuvenation: advances in diagnosis and treatment. JAMA Facial Plast Surg 2017;19:64–71.

30. Bellafill for acne scars. Med Lett Drugs Ther 2015; 57:93–4.

31. Cohen BE, Elbuluk N. Microneedling in skin of color: a review of uses and efficacy. J Am Acad Dermatol 2016;74:348–55.

32. Schulze R, Meehan KJ, Lopez A, et al. Low-fluence 1,064-nm laser hair reduction for pseudofolliculitis barbae in skin types IV, V, and VI. Dermatol Surg 2009;35:98–107.

33. Maranda EL, Simmons BJ, Nguyen AH, et al. Treatment of acne keloidalis nuchae: a systematic review of the literature. Dermatol Ther (Heidelb) 2016;6: 363–78.

Cosmeceuticals for Male Skin

Zoe Diana Draelos, MD[a,b],*

KEYWORDS

- Cosmeceuticals • Skin health • Antiaging • Male skin

KEY POINTS

- The male cosmeceutical market is interesting because most male cosmeceuticals are purchased by women and provided to their male counterparts.
- Male skin produces more sebaceous, eccrine, and apocrine secretions than female skin.
- Male skin functions differently from female skin in terms of not only cleansing to remove sebum and sweat but also skin moisturization needs.
- The best developed portion of the male skin care market is associated with facial hair removal known as shaving.

INTRODUCTION

The male cosmeceutical market is interesting because most male cosmeceuticals are purchased by women and provided to their male counterparts. This means that male cosmeceuticals must appeal to women for initial purchase but must also appeal to the men who use them on a daily basis. No one has yet cracked the male skin care market. Men have traditionally been uninterested in skin appearance, but this is changing generationally. Younger men are becoming increasingly more interested in fragrances, cleansers, and moisturizers. Aging is also become a concern, thus creating a desire to engage in the use of cosmeceuticals.

Cosmeceuticals are not recognized by the US Food and Drug Administration (FDA) from a regulatory standpoint. Cosmeceuticals are cosmetics and not drugs. They are purchased over the counter (OTC) and contain ingredients that are generally recognized as safe, requiring no regulation. Consumers know, however, that cosmeceuticals are cosmetic products that promise something more functionally relevant than just colored cosmetics. Male cosmeceuticals are distinct from female cosmeceuticals, because many of the products are aimed at addressing male facial hair. Preshave treatments, shaving products, and postshave skin care are unique to the male market, along with products designed to address increased male sebum, sweat, and the resulting body odor. There is also a perception that men must smell masculine whereas women should smell feminine. This category of male cosmeceuticals is the focus of this writing.

MALE SKIN VERSUS FEMALE SKIN CHARACTERISTICS

It may appear that male cosmeceuticals are the same as female cosmeceuticals, except for different packaging and fragrance. Products that are specifically designed for men must address more than just superficialities. Men have different skin care needs, as outlined in **Table 1**.

Men typically do not use colored cosmetics, such as powders and facial foundations because the beard does not allow an even film to be created over the cheeks. Men tend to have a darker skin

---

Disclosure: The author has nothing they wish to disclose.
[a] Department of Dermatology, Duke University School of Medicine, 40 Duke Medicine Circle, Durham, NC 27710, USA; [b] Private practice, Dermatology Consulting Services, 2444 North Main Street, High Point, NC 27262, USA
* Dermatology Consulting Services, 2444 North Main Street, High Point, NC 27262.
E-mail address: zdraelos@northstate.net

derm.theclinics.com

Table 1
Male and Female skin structure

Attribute	Female	Male
Skin color	Lighter	Darker
Red skin tones	Lower	Higher
Yellow skin tones	Higher	Lower
Skin thickness	Thinner	Thicker
Amount of collagen	Less	More
Rate of collagen loss	Same	Same
Subcutaneous fat	More	Less
Cellulite	More	Less
Appearance of aging	Faster	Slower

color than women, however, with different ratios of the pigments that create the appearance of healthy skin.[1] Male skin is darker than female skin, containing more melanin but also increased red tones from blood vessels and fewer yellow tones, probably due to less photoaging and thicker skin with more collagen.[2]

The male cosmeceutical market has never been as large as the female market, probably because men age more slowly than women. The facial hair is photoprotective and the thicker skin is less damaged by the deeply penetrating UV-A. Yet, women tend to have softer, smoother skin due the absence of less terminal hair and the presence of increased subcutaneous fat.[3] Although this might be an appearance blessing, it is also an appearance curse because it allows women to experience more cellulite than men.[4]

MALE SKIN CLEANSING NEEDS

Male skin produces more sebaceous, eccrine, and apocrine secretions than female skin. The sebaceous glands are larger and more abundant on male skin, especially on the face because they are tied to terminal hairs instead of the vellus hairs characteristic of the female face[5] (**Table 2**). This means male facial cleansers must be more

Table 2
Male and Female skin secretions

Attribute	Female	Male
Sebum production	Less	More
Sweat production	Less	More
Sweat evaporation rate	Higher	Lower
Body skin pH	Higher	Lower
Axilla skin pH	Same	Same

aggressive to remove sebum, which is why the male cleanser market is dominated by bar soap containing both soap and synthetic detergents, a formulation known as a combar. Syndet cleansers are also available in liquid forms, which are gaining traction in the male market, especially with the addition of male-oriented fragrances. High-impact fragrance body washes are becoming popular among younger men who use the cleanser to both clean and fragrance the skin. Body washes leave behind a fragrance due their emulsion characteristics. Although syndet is amphiphilic and binds the oil-soluble dirt for water rinsing, the lipid phase contains the fragrance and is left behind on the skin. Sebum removal is important on the male face and body to maintain the skin microbiome, which is rich in Propionibacterium *acnes*, accounting for face and back acne. The sebum also promotes the growth of *Malassezia restricta* and *Malassezia globosa*, fungal organisms responsible for seborrheic dermatitis. Thus, removing these organisms is important for the prevention of disease.

In addition to sebum issues, apocrine and eccrine sweat considerations are important. Men sweat more than women, making antiperspirants a common skin care product. The abundant sweat accompanied by a larger surface for bacterial growth due to body hair makes odor a larger issue for men than women.[6] Male-directed antiperspirants are also fragranced for the male preference and are characterized by a larger application surface for the larger male axilla. Technically antiperspirants are not cosmeceuticals but rather OTC drugs because they are regulated through an FDA monograph.

Increased male body odor, due to increased bacterial growth using sebum and sweat as a nutritional source, points to the need for the use of antibacterial cleansers. The most popular male antibacterial was triclosan, until 2016, when triclosan was removed from the market by the FDA. This led to the replacement of triclosan by benzalkonium chloride, which is the active ingredient in antibacterial liquid and bar cleansers. Especially in the armpit, male body odor is an issue. This use of antibacterial products to control this odor is a major cosmeceutical need; however, antibacterial products are also considered OTC drugs and are not technically cosmeceuticals.

MALE SKIN MOISTURIZATION

Male skin functions differently from female skin in terms of not only cleansing to remove sebum and sweat but also skin moisturization needs. Transepidermal water loss, the amount of water leaving the skin and entering the environment, is lower in women than men, even though polls show that women believe that their skin is drier. Women also generally believe that their skin sags more than men, but skin elasticity is identical between the genders. The increased impression of sagging may be due to thinning collagen rather than decreased skin elasticity.

Female skin is more biologically responsive than male skin. This is manifested by the lower temperature at which heat induces vasodilatation. It also presents as an increase in irritant contact dermatitis and increased sympathetic tone. This may explain why women exhibit increased redness and irritation to skin care products, sometimes referred to as sensitive skin, compared with men, who do not gravitate to sensitive skin product formulations.

Male skin moisturizers are a much smaller market than female-oriented moisturizers due to the sebum production drive of male-dominant testosterone.[7] Sebum provides skin moisturization, making the needs for facial and body creams for men somewhat different. Although men do develop dry skin at approximately age 60 years and older, dry skin is a much smaller male market. The male skin need for emolliency is greater due to smooth desquamating facial skin scale produced by shaving. Emollients fill the intercellular spaces where aggressive cleansing has removed the lipids to restore a smooth soft skin surface. The most popular emollient is dimethicone, which may be delivered to the skin surface in the form of a toner, aftershave lotion, skin bracer, or facial moisturizer. Toners are applied after cleansing, and aftershave lotions or skin bracers are applied after shaving. Toners can deliver a thin layer of dimethicone to decrease facial skin tightness. Aftershave lotions or skin bracers may contain a small amount of alcohol to decrease superficial bacterial infection and the papules/pustules associated with razor burn. In addition, the product can deliver some dimethicone emolliency to smooth skin scale and soothe irritated postshaving skin.

A new introduction in the male skin care market is moisturizers that are applied after shaving. These moisturizers have a lower viscosity designed to spread easily over the hair-bearing face. They may contain active ingredients, such as niacinamide, adapted from the female market, with the claim to increase epidermal turnover, improve skin pigmentation, and decrease skin irritation. Sometimes a sunscreen is included with a sun protection factor of between 15 and 30. These products still represent a minority of the male skin care market.

MALE ANTIAGING MOISTURIZERS

The antiaging moisturizer market is developing for men but very slowly. Because men do not age as quickly as women and periorbital wrinkles are considered masculine, antiaging moisturizers are not as popular in the male skin care market. The rugged coarse look is valued as a sign of masculinity and maturity. The thicker male skin is also less able to respond to beneficial effects of moisturization, especially on the hair-bearing upper cheeks.[8] Wrinkle creams simply do not have early appeal to men due to their perceived lack of need and poor immediate efficacy.

PHOTOPROTECTION

Some of the resistance of male skin to aging is due to the photoprotection afforded by facial hair. The follicle also increases skin thickness, decreasing the penetration of UV-A radiation into male skin. This allows women to age more rapidly than men, a phenomenon magnified by the media preference for younger leading women paired with older leading men. Thus, men do not see the need for the application of sun protection to same degree as their female counterparts.

SHAVING

The best developed portion of the male skin care market is associated with facial hair removal known as shaving. Shaving has an important impact on male facial skin care.[9] Shaving is the most effective physical facial exfoliation method, accounting for the lack of need to use exfoliating topical hydroxy acids, hand-held microdermabrasion devices, or mechanical brushes. The procedure efficiently removes desquamating corneocytes along with beard debris, obviating facials, peels, or other spa procedures. Shaving is also an effective method of removing open and closed comedones from the facial skin, making this activity a spa-type activity for men, improving skin smoothness, softness, and texture.

The newer flat razor designs are even more effective at improving skin appearance. These devices have multiple spring-mounted blades, decreasing razor burn and maintaining a steady angle, allowing the flat razor to glide over the skin surface, producing a closer shave without pressing the razor into the skin. This is accomplished by allowing the first blade to lift the hair, with each successive blade cutting the hairs closer and closer to the skin surface.

The success of a shave can also be improved by selecting a cosmeceutical shaving gel. The best designed cosmeceutical shaving products are the postforming shaving gels, which are dispensed as a gel and rubbed into the skin to form a foam, thereby enhancing water absorption into the hair, softening hair protein bonds, and decreasing the hair cutting force. It is said that a dry male beard hair shaft has the same resistance to cutting as a similar diameter copper wire whereas wet beard hair is softer, similar to an aluminum wire of similar diameter. The more water absorbed into the hair shaft, the softer the hair becomes and the closer the shave obtained.

REFERENCES

1. Fink B, Grammer K, Matts PJ. Visible skin color distribution plays a role in the perception of age, attractiveness, and health in female faces. Evol Hum Behav 2006;27(6):433–42.
2. Shuster S, Black MM, McVite E. The influence of age and sex on skin thickness, skin collagen and density. Br J Dermatol 1975;93(6):639–43.
3. Armstrong BK, Kricker A. The epidemiology of UV induced skin cancer. J Photochem Photobiol B 2001;63(1–3):8–18.
4. Mirrashed R, Sharp JC, Krause V, et al. Pilot study of dermal and subcutaneous fat structures by MRI in individuals who differ in gender, BMI, and cellulite grading. Skin Res Technol 2004;10(3):161–8.
5. Knip A. Measurement and regional distribution of functioning sweat glands in male and female Caucasians. Hum Biol 1969;41(3):380–7.
6. Leyden JJ, McGinley KJ, Holzle E, et al. The microbiology of the human axilla and its relationship to axillary odor. J Invest Dermatol 1981;77:413–6.
7. Imperato-McGinley J, Gautier T, Cai LQ, et al. The androgen control of sebum production. Studies of subjects with dihydrotestosterone deficiency and complete androgen insensitivity. J Clin Endocrinol Metab 1993;76(2):524–8.
8. Loden M. The clinical benefit of moisturizers. J Eur Acad Dermatol Venereol 2005;19(6):672–88.
9. Muscarella F. The evolutionary significance and social perception of male pattern baldness and facial hair. Ethol Sociobiol 1996;17(2):99–117.

Energy-Based Devices in Male Skin Rejuvenation

Margit Juhász, MD[a,b,*], Ellen Marmur, MD[a,c]

KEYWORDS

- Male • Aesthetics • Aging • Laser • Body contouring

KEY POINTS

- Men seek cosmetic procedures for vastly different reasons than women.
- Men often seek discrete cosmetic services with little downtime.
- Male skin structure generally differs from female skin structure.
- Dermatologists should consider subtle differences in the psyche of the male cosmetic patient.

INTRODUCTION

The age of the "Menaissance" has begun. With the incredible increase of male patients interested in the promise of "prejuvenation" and maintaining their "manity," nonsurgical cosmetic procedures using energy-based devices are increasingly popular.[1,2] This uptick can be attributed to the overall trend of highly accessible, safe, and minimally invasive cosmetic procedures for both men and women. Professional men switch jobs more than ever, and maintaining a youthful, productive, and energetic appearance has a high return on investment. Gone are the stigmas for men who seek cosmetic improvement, especially laser treatments.

Male grooming products alone have seen a yearly growth of 9%, with an estimated 29 billion USD spent by consumers in 2010.[1] The American Society of Aesthetic Plastic Surgeons (ASAPS) estimates that since 1997, there has been an increase by 325% in the number of cosmetic procedures performed on men, with 10.1% of total nonsurgical cosmetic procedures done on male patients and an estimated 12 billion USD worth of surgical and nonsurgical cosmetic procedures performed on men alone in 2014.[3,4] The National Ambulatory Medical Care Survey suggests, over the period of 1995 to 2003, that 21.3% of all nonsurgical cosmetic procedures were performed on male patients.[3] Most notably, the American Society for Dermatologic Surgery 2016 Survey on Dermatologic Procedures noted that the number of male cosmetic patients has greatly increased in the fields of both injectable neuromodulators (9% in the last 5 years) and soft tissue fillers (7% since 2015).[5] One small study originating in California stated that the most frequent aesthetic concerns for men included acne scars, poikiloderma, and telangiectasias.[1] In a survey of the top 5 nonsurgical procedures sought out by the male patient, laser hair removal and laser skin resurfacing rank second and fifth, respectively.[6]

It is important to note that men seek cosmetic procedures for vastly different reasons than women. Men want to regain their youthful appearance, because of their association of youth with power, being more competitive in the workplace, and success. The improvement in self-esteem, body image and subsequently, quality of life are just added benefits. To attain this rejuvenated look, men prefer to undergo small procedures with little downtime. In this regard, energy-based

Disclosure: The authors have no relevant conflicts of interest to disclose. The authors did not receive financial support for this research.

[a] Marmur Medical, 12 East 87th Street, Suite 1A, New York, NY 10128, USA; [b] Department of Dermatology, University of California, Irvine, 843 Health Sciences Road, Irvine, CA 92697, USA; [c] Department of Dermatology, Mount Sinai Hospital, 1 Gustave L Levy Place, New York, NY 10029, USA
* Corresponding author. Marmur Medical, 12 East 87th Street, Suite 1A, New York, NY 10128.
E-mail address: margit.lw.juhasz@gmail.com

devices appeal especially to male patients because of their efficacy, safety, and little to no downtime postprocedure (depending on which device is used).[4,7] Energy-based treatment options are often considered a "gateway" procedure for men and can lead to assessment for further, more invasive, procedures, such as injectables.[2]

According to an ASAPS survey that looked at nonsurgical cosmetic procedures performed during the period of 2005 to 2014, the procedures most performed on male patients were intense pulsed light (IPL) (13.9%) and then laser hair removal (12.9%).[3] Between the years of 2010 and 2014, it has been reported that the use of IPL has increased by 44%.[8] Male patients express interest in removing lentigines, seborrheic keratosis, poikiloderma, facial telangiectasias, deep rhytides, and neck laxity. Knowing which lasers and energy-based devices address these issues in the most time efficient ways is essential to treating male cosmetic patients.

SPECIAL CONSIDERATIONS IN THE MALE COSMETIC PATIENT SEEKING ENERGY-BASED SKIN REJUVENATION

Historically, men are often employed outdoors more frequently than women and therefore suffer from increased exposure to environmental insults, including UV radiation. This increased exposure to UV may explain why men have a higher incidence of skin cancer and increased induced-immunosuppression leading to greater subsequent mortality.[1,9] Often, men are less likely to practice sun-safe behavior, with 41% of men and boys never applying sunscreen. On average, men are more likely to be exposed to and partake in tobacco smoke, which has been shown to be an independent risk factor for cutaneous aging and elastosis.[9]

Male skin structure generally differs from female skin structure. Men's skin has an inherently thicker epidermal and dermal thickness due to increased hydroxyl-proline and collagen content. As men age and testosterone levels decrease, the epidermis and dermis also decrease in thickness. Male skin also exhibits decreased subcutaneous adipose tissue and increased skeletal muscle mass (including the face). A decrease in adipose tissue leads to flat and angular facial features. With the increase in facial memetic muscle mass, men often present with deeper expressive rhytides, except in the perioral area. These factors lead men to appear older when compared with women of the same age. An increase in androgen hormone leads to the development of coarse, pigmented terminal hairs of the face (chin and upper lip), trunk, and anterior thighs. Furthermore, men

have a larger dermal vascular plexus to provide blood flow to the increased amount of adnexal structures. In addition, male skin has an increased ceramide concentration, increased sebum levels, and increased sweat production as well as decreased pH and decreased vasodilatory properties.[1-3,9,10]

It is important to take note of these differences in the epidermal and dermal structure of men versus women. Increased skin thickness can cause increased scatter of a laser's photon beam, and therefore, higher fluences may need to be used in the male patient to achieve satisfactory results.[2,3] However, because of the increased vascularity, male patients are more prone to postprocedure erythema and bleeding complications, such as ecchymosis, especially in patients with rosacea or seborrheic dermatitis, and in the lower face. When using lasers, for purposes other than hair removal, it is important use these lasers carefully and appropriately to avoid iatrogenic alopecia in areas with terminal hairs (face, trunk).[9] In the authors' experience, because of the sheer number of terminal hairs in the beard and mustache distribution, permanent alopecia is rare. More commonly, telogen effluvium occurs in the treated areas and is self-resolving within 3 to 6 months. Finally, men have been shown to have slower wound healing and are more susceptible to skin infections after procedures.[8]

Dermatologists should consider subtle differences in the psyche of the male cosmetic patient. Unfortunately, until recently, literature suggested that a high percentage of men seeking cosmetic consultation had a psychiatric abnormality, including borderline personality and body dysmorphic disorder. However, the latest research refutes this claim as being simply not true. There may be a similar subset of male patients who have such personality disorders as there are female patients, and they must be consulted with care. Some reports suggest that men seek laser resurfacing treatment for acne scars more often than facial rejuvenation, compared with women who seek treatment for facial photo-aging more frequently. Although men would like to appear youthful and rejuvenated, they often do not want complete erasure of rhytides and other signs of aging. Instead, they often desire discretion and want their look "softened" with procedures that are less drastic, are minimally invasive, and require decreased postprocedure downtime.[3,8,11,12] Also, men are usually more hesitant, especially on their initial visit, to undergo multiple procedures at one time and often opt for a more conservative approach with one procedure at a time. In contrast to their reserved approach when receiving cosmetic procedures, male patients expect instant gratification with immediate results and no postprocedure side effects (such as erythema or edema).[3,8,11,12] Although they are less prone to acne flares after laser treatment, men (as discussed earlier) have a greater propensity for erythema and bruising after procedures because of their increased dermal vasculature. Men are also less likely to wear cover-up or make-up postprocedure, hence driving their wish for less invasive procedures[3,8,11,12] (Tables 1–3).

LIGHT-BASED AND LASER THERAPIES IN THE MALE PATIENT

Between the 1997 and 2014, laser procedures in male patients increased 9.4 times. Male patients often seek energy-based therapies for the treatment of acne scars, photodamage (including poikiloderma and rhytides), and complications of rosacea such as rhinophyma.[8] In a study comparing male to female patients seeking treatment with the erbium glass nonablative fractional laser, 44% of male patients seek treatment for acne scars, and 32% for photoaging; in comparison, 48% of female patients seek treatment for photoaging of the face, and 22% seek treatment for for photoaging of a nonface area.[2] As previously discussed, male cosmetic patients often favor minimally invasive procedures with less downtime postprocedure. Although research shows that ablative skin resurfacing has the most consistent improvement postprocedure, the

Table 1
Demographic data for the use of energy-based nonsurgical cosmetic data

Procedure	Female Patients (%)	Male Patients (%)
IPL	86.1	13.9
Laser hair removal	87.1	12.0
Fraxel	89.1	10.9
Noninvasive tightening	91.2	8.8
Ablative laser	93.5	6.5

Surveys done by The American Society for Aesthetic Plastic Surgery from 2005 to 2014 show that men are more likely to ask for minimally invasive procedures associated with little downtime (IPL, hair removal) versus more invasive ablative laser therapy, unlike female patients.
Data from The American Society for Aesthetic Plastic Surgery. Procedure surveys from 2005 to 2014. Available at: https://www.surgery.org/media/. Accessed October 4, 2017; and *From* Frucht CS, Ortiz AE. Nonsurgical cosmetic procedures for men: trends and technique considerations. J Clin Aesthet Dermatol 2016;9(12):33–43.

Table 2
Demographic data for the use of energy-based nonsurgical cosmetic data

Procedure	Female Patients (%)	Male Patients (%)
Laser hair removal	84.9	15.1
Resurfacing (CO_2 laser, chemical peel, dermabrasion)	88.3	11.7
Nonablative rejuvenation	93.6	6.4

These data derived from The International Society of Aesthetic Plastic Surgery procedure survey in 2013 echo the ASAPS survey with men favoring procedures such as a hair removal.
Data from The International Society of Aesthetic Plastic Surgery. ISAPS International Survey on Aesthetic/Cosmetic Procedures Performed in 2013. Available at: https://www.isaps.org/Media/Default/globalstatistics/2014%20ISAPS%20Results%20(3).pdf. Accessed October 4, 2017; and *From* Frucht CS, Ortiz AE. Nonsurgical cosmetic procedures for men: trends and technique considerations. J Clin Aesthet Dermatol 2016;9(12):33–43.

man's wish for discretion may lead them to choose IPL, and nonablative and fractional ablative treatments. As with all patients, it is especially important to provide written instructions for pretreatments and posttreatments, realistic expectations, and exactly when treatment should be done to male patients. Explain concisely that these treatment options may require multiple sessions, and improvement may be small in comparison to ablative resurfacing.[8]

In the authors' experience, male laser consultations differ from consultations with most female patients. Many men have less experience with and less clinical knowledge about laser procedures. They have not read extensively about the different options and have fewer questions. The visit may seem like the quickest consultation

Table 3
Men and women seek nonablative fractional resurfacing treatment for different reasons

Top 3 Reasons Men Seek Laser Resurfacing	Top 3 Reasons Women Seek Laser Resurfacing
Acne scars	Facial photo-aging
Facial photo-aging	Nonfacial photo-aging
Traumatic/surgical scars	Acne scars

Data from Frucht CS, Ortiz AE. Nonsurgical cosmetic procedures for men: trends and technique considerations. J Clin Aesthet Dermatol 2016;9(12):36.

ever, but take time to explain the general principle of each laser, how it works (eg, selective photothermolysis for superficial pigment using a specific wavelength), the pain level, and the downtime. Written information should be provided as well as contact information for questions postprocedure to ensure a successful experience for all parties.

Facial Resurfacing

Fully ablative lasers include the CO_2 and erbium:yttrium-aluminum-garnet (Er:YAG), which target water as their chromophore. Fully ablative laser resurfacing is excellent for rhinophyma, deep rhytides, poikiloderma of the face, and acne scarring. As the most powerful laser treatment, ablative resurfacing may not be the first option suggested to the male patient. Resurfacing with ablative lasers has increased complications, including erythema, edema, bruising, crusting, reactivation of herpes, infection, scarring, and pigmentary changes. Pretreatment with antibiotics, antivirals, sun protection, targeted cosmeceuticals and review of explicit posttreatment instructions greatly reduces complications. Because men do not often want to wear cosmetics to cover unsightly postprocedure effects, or they do not have adequate downtime for recovery, they may not select these procedures even though these lasers are very effective.[12] One option is to offer mild to medium ablative treatments with a quicker recovery time at slightly more frequent intervals for optimal results.

Another excellent option is fractional laser resurfacing. Fractional technology has become increasingly popular because it treats the skin a fraction at a time, creating thousands of microthermal treatment zones without stripping the entire epidermis. As the epidermis is not ablated, fractionated lasers allow for faster repair and regeneration, with decreased side effects and downtime after treatment. These properties make fractionated laser treatment a more attractive option for male patients, and surveys show that fractional systems are increasing in popularity.[5,12] Fractional ablative lasers are extremely effective at treating laxity, photodamage, and scarring, but in some patients, the results are modest in comparison to fully ablative laser.

In a small study using fractionated ablative CO_2 laser (10,600 nm) for facial resurfacing, at 30 W with 500-μm pitch for 1000 μs to 1500 μs, male patients comprised 13.3% of the subjects enrolled. All patients were of Fitzpatrick skin type I to III. Patients were subjected to 2 to 3 treatment sessions at 8-week intervals. After treatment, all patients reported a mean improvement of 48.5% (including

skin texture, skin laxity, dyschromia, and global cosmetic outcome). Adverse events reported were minimal (pinpoint bleeding, edema, erythema, crusting, and bronzing) and lasted a maximum of 1 week before spontaneously resolving. There were no reports of scarring, postprocedure changes in pigmentation, or superficial infection.[13] Another fractionated laser system is erbium-based (Fraxel laser; Solta Medical Inc., Hayward, CA, USA). Treatment guidelines in the male patient include 6 mJ to 12 mJ superficial pigmented lesions can be treated; 10 mJ to 20 mJ for fine wrinkles; and 25 mJ to 40 mJ for deeper rhytides and scarring. In a study using Fraxel, researchers found that 8 to 10 passes over regions of mild to moderate atrophic acne scars showed significant posttreatment improvement in all patients.[12]

Intense pulse light (IPL) and broad band light (BBL) are extremely popular noninvasive cosmetic treatment options in the male population. IPL and BBL are essentially the same technology. IPL and BBL are used for the treatment of irregular skin pigmentation, rhytides, unwanted hair, as well as telangiectasias. There have been no studies focusing on the use of IPL/BBL exclusively in the male patient; however, multiple studies have looked at the efficacy of IPL/BBL treatment of a variety of skin abnormalities in a female or mixed patient population. For skin rejuvenation, multiple studies have reported anywhere from 60% to 90% improvement in skin texture, pigmentation, and telangiectasia. The most commonly reported side effects are erythema, hyperpigmentation or hypopigmentation, and blistering/crusting at the site of treatment.[14]

The scalp is an overlooked area of male photodamage. In men affected by alopecia, the scalp becomes more exposed to UV radiation causing lentigines, rhytides, and keratoses and thus contributes to a more aged appearance. A small study used nonablative fractional thulium fiber laser (1927 nm) on 4 male patients, ages 45 to 67 years, with extensive photo-damage and Fitzpatrick skin type II to III; 2 of the patients had previously undergone photodynamic therapy for actinic keratoses (AKs) of the scalp. Patients received topical anesthesia followed by laser treatment with a fluence of 20 mJ, 70% coverage, treatment level 11, with 8 passes for a total energy of 3.30 kJ. Two weeks after treatment, this study reported a 60% to 90% improvement in dyschromia (including hyperpigmentation), solar lentigines, and seborrheic keratoses. The patients tolerated the procedure well, and side effects were minimal with erythema, edema, and crusting that spontaneously resolved in 7 to 10 days.[15] Although this is just one study, it emphasizes the importance of aggressive laser settings when treating areas of male skin that have an increased thickness and high sebaceous content. In addition, with an increase in the male "Baby Boomer" population, rejuvenation of the scalp may become an increasingly popular cosmetic procedure.

In those male patients who want to avoid the supposed "stigma" of cosmetic procedures, photodynamic therapy with aminolevulinic acid combined with blue light therapy for the treatment of AKs has previously be shown to be beneficial for other signs of photodamage, including dyschromia and rhytides. In addition, one can also suggest the use of light or laser therapies (such as the 1927-nm thulium laser) for the treatment of AKs with the happy coincidence that these also treat concurrent signs of sun damage.[2]

Rhinophyma

Rhinophyma represents the end stage of rosacea, presenting as erythematous, bulbous enlargement of the nose, and can be associated with nasal outflow obstruction. This condition affects exclusively Caucasian men. Although electrocautery, cryosurgery, dermabrasion, and surgical excision have all been used as treatment modalities, ablative CO_2 and erbium laser resurfacing are popular options.[2] One study reports the use of CO_2 laser to delineate the area of correction (5 W, focused to 1 mm) and then to penetrate the skin by approximately 0.5 mm (15 W, focused to 3 mm) to sculpt hypertrophied regions. Another group used 4 passes of dual-mode Er:YAG (3-mm spot, 100-μm ablation) with excellent cosmetic outcome. In addition to resurfacing, these lasers may also be used for homeostasis after surgical excision of the rhinophyma.[12] Unfortunately, there have been no head-to-head studies comparing the CO_2 versus erbium laser as the primary treatment of rhinophyma. Anecdotally, though, dermatologists report that the Er:YAG laser results in less nonspecific tissue damage compared with CO_2 laser therapy.[12]

Tattoo Removal

Given the difference in the skin anatomy of men versus women, there may be a discrepancy in response to laser tattoo removal. The thicker epidermis and dermis of male patients may cause increased photo scattering, and therefore, less energy directed at the chromophore of choice. Using a q-switched 1064/532-nm Nd:YAG or q-switched 755-nm alexandrite laser, researchers showed that only 42.2% of male patients achieved tattoo clearance in comparison to 53.7% of female patients after 10 treatment sessions. Other factors that decreased the efficacy of tattoo removal

included larger size (>30 cm^2), high color density, non-red or non-black pigments, lower extremity location, shorter treatment intervals, and smoking.[2] New picoseconds lasers and also fractional energy devices make tattoo removal much more successful.

Laser Hair Removal

Laser hair removal is the second most common cosmetic procedure in the male patient. Commonly used devices for laser hair removal include the 1064-nm neodymium-doped yttrium aluminum garnet (Nd:YAG) as well as the 810-nm diode, 694-nm long-pulsed ruby, and 755-nm long-pulsed alexandrite. The Nd:YAG is considered the most effective with minimal side effects, including erythema, purpura, and folliculitis. The Nd:YAG may also be used safely in darker Fitzpatrick skin types with less concern for dyschromia. It is important to be careful with the fluence level used during treatment, because aggressive treatment may result in surrounding melanin targeting and subsequent changes in skin pigmentation postprocedure.[2,8] In addition to cosmetic reasons, men may also require laser hair removal for pseudofolliculitis barbae (PFB). In these cases, the Nd:YAG has been shown to be an effective therapeutic option. In one study, 3 months after treatment (50–100 J/cm^2, 5-mm spot, 50-ms pulse), patients exhibited a significant decreased in PFB papules. Another study reported an 83% improvement from baseline with treatment (12 J/cm^2, 10-mm spot, 20-ms pulse).[2]

Genitalia

The face and scalp happen not to be the only area of concern when it comes to male skin rejuvenation. Pearly penile papules (PPP) affect anywhere from 14.3% to 48% of the male population. These flesh-colored, dome-shaped, less than 3-mm papules are located at the base of the glans and are completely benign. However, these papules often cause great psychological distress to the male patient. Treatment options for PPP previously included circumcision, podophyllin, cryotherapy, or electrodessication and curettage; often these procedures are uncomfortable for the patient and may leave adverse cosmetic outcomes (including changes in skin pigmentation, scarring, and disfigurement). Various laser modalities have been used for removal, including CO_2 laser (100–22,000 mJ/cm^2 for 1 to 2 treatment sessions), pulsed dye laser (600–1000 mJ/cm^2 for 1 to 3 treatment sessions), and fractional photothermolysis (1550 nm for 5 sessions), with the most commonly used being the Er:YAG laser (400–500 mJ/cm^2 for 2 treatment sessions). All 55 cases reported in the literature reported complete clearance of the papules after treatment with minimal side effects postprocedure, and no reports of scarring or dyspigmentation.[16] Current data, although limited, show that laser therapy may be a good tool for the treatment of PPP without major adverse events. However, the body of literature on this subject is small, and further studies will need to be completed to determine long-term efficacy and safety.

Avoiding Erythema and Edema Postprocedure

To avoid complications of laser and light-based therapies, several anecdotal techniques have been suggested to reduce postprocedure erythema and edema. One suggestion is to use a 590-nm LED after nonablative laser treatment to minimize downtime post-photorejuvenation. Another suggestion is one-time application of a high-potency topical corticosteroid immediately after laser treatment. These techniques have yet to be properly studied in a controlled setting.[2,3]

THE USE OF RADIOFREQUENCY DEVICES FOR FACIAL REJUVENATION

Multiple types of radiofrequency (RF) modalities exist: monopolar, bipolar, tripolar, multipolar, and multigenerator. These technologies are based on turning RF energy into thermal energy directed at dermal collagen bundles, thus causing collagen destruction, remodeling, and neocollagenesis. RF does not target specific chromophores in the skin and therefore anecdotally has been shown to be safer in darker skin types because the risks of pigmentary changes posttreatment are minimal. In addition, side effects, such as erythema, crusting, and blisters, are minimal, making RF an appealing choice for the male cosmetic patient. By combining RF with other rejuvenation modalities (such as vacuum, light sources, and microneedling), dermatologists can exploit a diverse field of devices for anesthetic rejuvenation especially for correcting facial and neck skin laxity.[17,18]

In addition to multiple modalities of RF, new technology has been applied to RF devices to allow for increasing results with decreased side effects. Using "fractional" technology from laser devices, fractionated RF demonstrates significant neocollagenesis and neoelastogenesis on histology posttreatment; most likely areas of tissue unaffected by the RF tissue provide reservoirs of cytokines and growth factors to allow for rapid remodeling of affected areas. Temperature-controlled RF devices provide precise administration of heat energy to the dermal and subdermal layers using an internal thermistor to accurately monitor subdermal temperatures and a thermal camera to monitor the epidermal temperature.[18] These devices ensure adequate heating of the dermal layers of collagen, while minimizing thermal damage to the epidermis. Although no studies have been completed on RF for cosmetic purposes exclusively in the male patient, results from prior studies in female and mixed patient populations may be extrapolated.[12]

Plasma skin resurfacing or rejuvenation (PSR) has been shown to increase collagen remodeling and is useful for the treatment of rhytides and dyschromia. Because of the precise heating of targeted tissue, PSR results in minimal injury of the surrounding areas. Because this treatment option is not associated with dyspigmentation postprocedure, it is ideal for patients with Fitzpatrick skin types IV–VI who may develop postinflammatory hyperpigmentation or hypopigmentation after laser treatment.[12] Coblation is based on bipolar RF technology and is an ablative technology resulting in epidermal exfoliation. As with all ablative methods, coblation is effective for the treatment of photoaging (dyschromia, skin laxity), rosacea (telangiectasias), and scarring. Because of the risk of pigmentary changes posttreatment, this method is also not recommended for darker skin types. Bipolar RF has been combined with other nonablative technologies to maximize the benefits of ablative technology, while trying to minimize adverse events and downtime; examples include RF and IPL, RF and infrared light, or RF and diode laser.[12]

MICRONEEDLING IN THE MALE PATIENT

Microneedling has become a popular method of skin rejuvenation. Because it is not laser-based, there is little damage to melanocytes and therefore less risk of pigmentary changes postprocedure. At about age 40 to 50 years old, male skin hydration decreases. Using a stamp microneedle combined with automated 0.020-mL intradermal noncrosslinked hyaluronic acid injections (Dermashine Balance, Huons Co., Ltd., Seongnam, South Korea and Elravie Balance, Humidex Co., Ltd., Anyang, South Korea), a small study found that 3 treatment sessions at 2-week intervals in 6 East Asian male patients resulted in increased skin hydration (measured by corneometry) up to 12 weeks after the final treatment and decreased transepidermal water loss up to 4 weeks posttreatment. Researchers did not find a significant improvement in skin elasticity. The patients enrolled were highly satisfied with their outcomes and all rated their improvement as "much improved" to "very much improved" on the Global Aesthetic Improvement Scale (GAIS). Side effects were minor and reported as pain and mild erythema.[19]

BODY CONTOURING USING ENERGY DEVICES IN THE MALE PATIENT

Male patients are increasingly seeking surgical and nonsurgical body contouring to obtain slimmer and more svelte figures, with special attention to the abdominal region; body contouring procedures have increased from 32.9% in 2005 to 64% as of 2013, as well as a reported 158% increase between the years of 2012 and 2014. The 2 most common surgical procedures reported in the male patient population are breast reduction and liposuction. However, noninvasive procedures for skin tightening and fat reduction are growing in popularity with almost 6 times as many nonsurgical procedures completed compared with surgical procedures. Again, as mentioned previously, men may prefer noninvasive body contouring procedures because of the discretion, minimal downtime, and few postprocedure complications.[8,20]

Arguably, one of the most popular noninvasive body-sculpting techniques is cryolipolysis (Cool-Sculpting; Zeltiq Aesthetics Inc., Pleasanton, CA, USA), a technology that exploits the fact that adipocytes are more sensitive to cold temperatures than the surrounding tissue. Studies using cryolipolysis in the male patient have shown a 20.4% reduction in subcutaneous fat at 2 months (which equals about an average of 56 mL of volume loss), which increased to 25.5% at 6 months posttreatment. In patient surveys, 86% report noticeable subjective improvement in treatment areas and 73% of patients report being satisfied with their results. Although abdomen, back, and flanks have been reported as the most successful areas for treatment, pseudo-gynecomastia has also been treated with cryolipolysis. After 2 sessions spaced 2 months apart, researchers demonstrated a 1.6-mm reduction in fat tissue by ultrasound (US); 95% of patients reported being satisfied with their results.[8,20] It is important to note that the side effect of paradoxical adipocyte hyperplasia (PAH) is more commonly reported in the male cosmetic patient population than female patients. It is estimated that PAH occurs in 0.021% of treatments worldwide, and of these, 55% of cases involve male patients. Although the direct mechanism has not yet been elucidated, researchers hypothesize that sexual dimorphism of adipose tissue anatomy may be a key factor. For instance, male adipose tissue is often located viscerally, has an increased amount of parallel placed fibrous septa, and may have a higher rate of mechanotransduction (a process in which low-level mechanical stress is converted into biochemical signals, inducing cytoskeletal reorganization and cellular growth). Therefore, it is important to choose male patients carefully and ensure they are without visceral fat deposits or fibrous, firm adipose tissue to avoid this unwanted adverse event.[8,20,21]

Several studies, which included male subjects, have been completed using US for adipose tissue reduction. In male patients, researchers have studied the use of US (UltraShape; UltraShape Ltd., Yokne'am, Isreal and Liposonix, Medicis Technologies Corp., Bothell, WA, USA) for pseudo-gynecomastia, as well as thigh and abdominal contouring. Although studies have not been completed using exclusively male subjects, US-assisted circumference reduction has been shown to be anywhere from 1.9 to 4.6 cm. Side effects are usually mild and self-limiting, ranging from erythema to blistering, as well as alterations in sensation.[20] Low-level light therapy (LLLT) is another contouring technique that has been studied in male patients. Using LLLT devices (Zerona LipoLaser, Erchonia Medical, Inc., McKinney, TX, USA and Meridian LAPEX 2000 LipoLaser System, Meridian Medical, Inc., White Rock, BC, Canada), researchers have demonstrated an average of 13.1-cm decrease in circumference from the abdomen and hip/thigh regions.[20] Although RF has yet to be studied in male patients, multiple studies have been completed using female subjects. In prior studies on women, RF has been shown to decrease abdominal circumference by 4.45%, equaling anywhere from a 1.82-cm to 4.93-cm average circumferential reduction. The most commonly reported side effect is self-resolving erythema.[20] It may be possible in the future to combine various noninvasive body sculpting techniques (cryolipolysis, RF, and HIFU) to create synergistic results and even more adipose tissue reduction.

In the recent years, advances in liposuction technique and technology have allowed for the introduction of laser-assisted liposuction (LAL). By introducing an optic fiber (1064-nm Nd:YAG or 980-nm diode laser) encased within the microcannula, LAL allows for thermal elimination of adipose tissue. This technique has been studied in fat reduction of head and neck areas as well as for gynecomastia. With LAL, gynecomastia reduction can be as large as 50%. Histologic studies have shown that LAL may also induce neocollagenesis, thereby reducing excess skin after adipose tissue destruction. Because of the use of direct thermal energy and subsequent coagulation, there is reduced blood loss and hematoma formation in the more vascular dermis of male patients.[8,22]

SUMMARY

Dermatologists practicing in the Menaissance era are intrigued to understand the complexities of the male cosmetic patient. Men are a rapidly growing but untapped patient population. With shifts in societal norms and traditional paradigms of the masculine identity, as well as the social de-stigmatization of men obtaining cosmetic procedures, male patients are now seeking consultation for cosmetic enhancement and rejuvenation.

It is easy to assume that your male patients want and require the same services as female patients; however, multiple studies have shown that men approach noninvasive cosmetic procedures in a vastly different manner compared with women. Men often seek discrete cosmetic services with little downtime. It is here that energy-based technologies find their niche in the cosmetic male patient. Being often minimally invasive, with few posttreatment side effects, these procedures are attractive to the male patient. However, one must also be ready subsequently to address any expectation-performance mismatches that result from these treatments.

Unfortunately, data are lacking specifically on minimally invasive cosmetic procedures in the male population. Most procedures, including energy-based techniques, are performed in men based on either anecdotal evidence or information garnered from studies in female patients. Because there are significant differences in the anatomy of the epidermis and dermis in male versus female patients, more research will need to be completed regarding energy-based technologies in the male patient to provide evidence-based guidelines for treatment. In the meantime, energy-based male rejuvenation is an exciting challenge and will certainly lead to new techniques and technologies that will benefit our patients.

REFERENCES

1. Elsner P. Overview and trends in male grooming. Br J Dermatol 2012;166(Suppl 1):2–5.
2. Green JB, Metelitsa AI, Kaufman J, et al. Laser and light-based aesthetics in men. J Drugs Dermatol 2015;14(9):1061–4.
3. Frucht CS, Ortiz AE. Nonsurgical cosmetic procedures for men: trends and technique considerations. J Clin Aesthet Dermatol 2016;9(12):33–43.
4. Rieder EA, Mu EW, Brauer JA. Men and cosmetics: social and psychological trends of an emerging demographic. J Drugs Dermatol 2015;14(9):1023–6.
5. ASDS. American Society for Dermatology Surgery (ASDS) Survey on Dermatologic Procedures 2016. 2017.
6. Werschler WP. Cosmetic dermatology in the male patient. Dermatol Ther 2007;20:377–8.
7. Fried RG. Esthetic treatment modalities in men: psychologic aspects of male cosmetic patients. Dermatol Ther 2007;20(6):379–84.
8. Cohen BE, Bashey S, Wysong A. Literature review of cosmetic procedures in men: approaches and techniques are gender specific. Am J Clin Dermatol 2017;18(1):87–96.
9. Keaney T. Male aesthetics. Skin Therapy Lett 2015;20(2):5–7.
10. Keaney TC. Aging in the male face: intrinsic and extrinsic factors. Dermatol Surg 2016;42(7):797–803.
11. Daines SM, Mobley SR. Considerations in male aging face consultation: psychologic aspects. Facial Plast Surg Clin North Am 2008;16(3):281–7, v.
12. Poore SO, Shama L, Marcus B. Facial resurfacing of the male patient. Facial Plast Surg Clin North Am 2008;16(3):357–69, vii.
13. Tierney EP, Hanke CW. Fractionated carbon dioxide laser treatment of photoaging: prospective study in 45 patients and review of the literature. Dermatol Surg 2011;37(9):1279–90.
14. Fodor L, Carmi N, Fodor A, et al. Intense pulsed light for skin rejuvenation, hair removal, and vascular lesions: a patient satisfaction study and review of the literature. Ann Plast Surg 2009;62(4):345–9.
15. Boen M, Wilson MJ, Goldman MP, et al. Rejuvenation of the male scalp using 1,927 nm non-ablative fractional thulium fiber laser. Lasers Surg Med 2017;49(5):475–9.
16. Maranda EL, Akintilo L, Hundley K, et al. Laser therapy for the treatment of pearly penile papules. Lasers Med Sci 2017;32(1):243–8.
17. Sadick N, Rothaus KO. Aesthetic applications of radiofrequency devices. Clin Plast Surg 2016;43(3):557–65.
18. Sadick N, Rothaus KO. Minimally invasive radiofrequency devices. Clin Plast Surg 2016;43(3):567–75.
19. Seok J, Hong JY, Choi SY, et al. A potential relationship between skin hydration and stamp-type microneedle intradermal hyaluronic acid injection in middle-aged male face. J Cosmet Dermatol 2016;15(4):578–82.
20. Singh B, Keaney T, Rossi AM. Male body contouring. J Drugs Dermatol 2015;14(9):1052–9.
21. Keaney TC, Naga LI. Men at risk for paradoxical adipose hyperplasia after cryolipolysis. J Cosmet Dermatol 2016;15(4):575–7.
22. Wollina U, Goldman A. Minimally invasive esthetic procedures of the male breast. J Cosmet Dermatol 2011;10(2):150–5.

The Use of Neurotoxins in the Male Face

Isabela T. Jones, MD[a],*, Sabrina G. Fabi, MD[b,c]

KEYWORDS

- Male aesthetics • Botulinum toxin • Male • Injections • Sex factors • Facial muscles

KEY POINTS

- Men have unique aesthetic goals, expectations, facial anatomy, and aging processes and thus require a tailored approach to botulinum toxin injections.
- Men have more skeletal muscle mass and produce greater facial movements than women and thus generally require a higher number of units of botulinum toxin.
- Approaches for the upper face are better supported by literature than for the lower face, but more studies are needed to further investigate gender differences.

INTRODUCTION

Injection of neurotoxin remains the most commonly performed cosmetic procedure in the United States, with 7.1 million cases being performed in 2016.[1] Although men have consistently comprised 6% of the proportion of these patients, the total number has grown by 355% since the year 2000, with 428,542 injections of neurotoxin being performed in men in the year 2015.[2] Because of this increase, providers have become more cognizant of the need to tailor their consultation and injection technique to male patients. Men have unique goals, expectations, facial anatomy, and aging processes. However, few clinical studies have evaluated gender differences in botulinum toxin dosing, technique, efficacy, and safety. This article serves as a guide for practitioners who provide injectable neurotoxins to men.

GOALS AND EXPECTATIONS IN MALE PATIENTS

Men generally seek cosmetic procedures in order to appear youthful. In an online survey of 600 men aged 30 to 65 years, Jagdeo and colleagues[3] found the main reason respondents would consider a facial injectable were to look good for their age and to look more youthful. Another survey, conducted by the American Academy of Facial Plastic and Reconstructive Surgery, showed that "looking younger, work-related concerns," and wanting to improve competitiveness were the main reasons men pursued cosmetic procedures.[4] Because it is minimally invasive and requires no down time, botulinum toxin is an especially attractive procedure for men who wish to appear more youthful.

The pretreatment consultation is essential in preparing for a successful outcome and satisfied patient. Some men come in for a particular concern or are seeking enhancement, whereas others desire a general antiaging consultation. Therefore, it is important to ascertain the patient's concerns and aesthetic goals. A physical examination should also be performed during the visit, assessing the patient from frontal and oblique views at rest and during facial expression, taking note of baseline asymmetries, presence of static

Disclosures: S.G. Fabi is a consultant and researcher for Allergan, Merz Pharmaceuticals, Galderma, and Revance. I.T. Jones has nothing to disclose.

[a] McLean Dermatology and Skincare Center, McLean, VA, USA; [b] Cosmetic Laser Dermatology, Goldman, Butterwick, Groff, Fabi & Wu, a West Dermatology Company, 9339 Genesee Avenue, Suite 300, San Diego, CA 92121, USA; [c] Department of Dermatology, University of California San Diego, 8899 University Center Lane, San Diego, CA 92122, USA

* Corresponding author. 6849 Old Dominion Drive Suite 340, McLean, VA 22101

E-mail address: isabelatjones@gmail.com

derm.theclinics.com

and dynamic rhytides, and muscle mass. In addition, educate the patient on the recommended procedures, possible adverse events, and expectations. Explain that there is increased patient satisfaction with continued retreatment, and that although dynamic rhytides are most responsive, static lines can improve with repeated injection.[5] Also, review interventions other than botulinum toxin that may be necessary to achieve optimal results, such as fillers, lasers, skin-tightening procedures, chemical or cold lipolysis, and surgery.

It is important to advise patients on common side effects, like transient edema, erythema, and bruising. Men specifically may be more likely to develop ecchymoses. Men undergoing facial plastic surgery have a higher incidence of postoperative hematoma,[6] which may be explained by the findings that, on the face, men have higher blood vessel density, more microvessels, increased perfusion via Doppler, and larger hair follicles.[7–9] In our practice, we use a 0.3-mL BD syringe with a 31-gauge, 8-mm needle (Becton Dickinson Labware, Franklin Lakes, NJ). For sensitive patients, a 32-gauge needle can provide more comfort than a 30-gauge needle.[10]

BOTULINUM TOXIN TYPES

Botulinum toxin is produced by *Clostridium botulinum*, an anaerobic, gram-positive, spore-forming rod. The bacterium produces 8 distinguishable neurotoxins. Although both types A and B are currently US Food and Drug Administration (FDA) approved, only type A toxin has indications for cosmetic use (**Table 1**). The toxin is composed of a 100-kDa heavy chain and a 50-kDa light chain, linked by a disulfide bridge.[11] The heavy chain binds the presynaptic neuron, allowing entry of the light chain into the cytoplasm. The light chain in turn binds and deactivates a component of the soluble *N*-ethylmaleimide–sensitive factor attachment protein receptor (SNARE) complex. A functioning SNARE complex is needed to release stored acetylcholine from the presynaptic neuron. Botulinum toxin types A and B have different targets within the SNARE complex.[12]

Aside from a unique mechanism of action, each commercially available type of neurotoxin has unique composition, complexing proteins, manufacturing, dosing, and clinical efficacy. Products are available in different vial sizes and can be reconstituted to various concentrations. Because of these dissimilarities, there is no standardized dose-response equivalence between different botulinum toxin products. The area of diffusion of botulinum toxin widens with increasing volume and concentration. Studies have shown that the field effect (action halo on muscular and sweat gland activity) is comparable among the various products if using equal volumes and equipotent doses.[13] The approximate dose conversions in **Table 1** have been obtained from experimental studies and consensus guidelines.[13–17] For the remainder of this article, recommended doses are based on onabotulinumtoxinA (OBA), unless otherwise specified.

Although the body of literature comparing different botulinum toxin types is growing, the study

Table 1
Botulinum neurotoxin type A

Generic Name	OnabotulinumtoxinA	AbobotulinumtoxinA	IncobotulinumtoxinA
Brand Name	Botox (Botox Cosmetic, Allergan, Irvine, CA)	Dysport (Galderma Pharma SA, Lausanne, Switzerland)	Xeomin (Merz Pharmaceuticals, Frankfurt, Germany)
Mechanism	Synaptosomal-associated protein 25 (SNAP-25)	SNAP-25	SNAP-25
Aesthetic FDA Indications (Approval Year)	Glabella (2002) Lateral canthal lines (2013) Forehead lines (2017)	Glabella (2009)	Glabella (2011)
Vial Sizes	50 U 100 U	300 U	100 U
Reconstitution Volume (Concentration)	2.5 mL for 100 U vial (4 U/0.1 mL)	3.0 mL (10 U/0.1 mL)	2.5 mL for 100 U vial (4 U/0.1 mL)
Relative Strength (OnabotulinumtoxinA/Product)	1:1	1:2–1:3 (likely closer to 1:2)	1:1

of gender differences in response to botulinum remains sparse. Only 3 studies have examined male-specific dosing, all to the glabella.[18–20] Although the specifics of each study are discussed later, they support the use of greater botulinum toxin doses in men, which is likely because men have a greater muscle mass. Studies have shown that men have a greater skeletal muscle mass, influenced by the anabolic effect of androgens.[21,22] In addition, men produce greater facial muscle movements.[23,24] The findings that men have greater muscle mass and facial movements supports the suggestion that men need higher doses of botulinum toxin than women to achieve comparable results. Nevertheless, not all male patients and treatment areas require higher doses. In some instances, the goal may be to reduce rather than eliminate muscle activity. This article discusses the aesthetic use of botulinum toxin in male patients by location on the face and neck, pointing out gender-specific differences in anatomy, goals, dosing, and injection technique.

UPPER FACE
Forehead

Neurotoxin can be used in the frontalis muscle to decrease the presence of transverse forehead lines. In their online survey, Jagdeo and colleagues[3] found that the forehead is the third most likely area to receive treatment in male patients.

Anatomy
The frontalis muscle is the only brow elevator. The muscle originates from the galea aponeurotica in the scalp, and inserts into the subcutaneous tissue and deep dermis above the superciliary arch.[25] Some fibers interdigitate with the corrugator supercilii, procerus, and orbicularis oculi muscles. Compared with women, the forehead in men has a greater height and width.[26] In addition, the presence of androgenetic alopecia further increases the height of the forehead. There are also differences in brow shape and location: the male brow is straighter, more horizontal, and sits lower on the orbital rim.[27] A Japanese study examining the facial wrinkles of 173 men and women aged 21 to 75 years showed that men had more severe forehead lines than women at all ages.[28]

Treatment goals
Although neurotoxin can completely immobilize the forehead, goals must be discussed with the patient. The presence of rhytides can impart a more distinguished appearance to the male face. Therefore, softening the horizontal lines while still allowing some movement is often preferred in men. In addition, the position and shape of the

brow is of utmost importance when discussing aesthetic goals. An arched brow can feminize the male face, whereas a brow that sits too low can interfere with vision, cause a heavy sensation, and impart an aged and antagonistic appearance.

Dosing and injection technique

- The consensus recommendations for the forehead are a total of 8 to 25 units, placing 2 to 4 units in 4 to 8 injection points (**Fig. 1**).[29]
- Injections are best placed intramuscularly in horizontal rows, with purposeful injection of the lateral frontalis in order to prevent arching of the brow. However, in men with lower-set eyebrows, keep the injection points higher on the frontalis to prevent excessive heaviness of the brow. Some experts use a lower dose per unit volume for injections into the dermis in the lower frontalis, because they believe this technique can improve rhytides in the lower forehead without causing brow descent.[29]
- Staying at least 1 cm above the orbital rim avoids diffusion of neurotoxin into the levator palpebrae superioris, which can result in upper eyelid ptosis.
- In men with androgenetic alopecia, also place injection points on the frontal scalp to prevent an unnatural wrinkling in this area (**Fig. 2**).

Glabella

Men tend to have a deeper furrow in the glabella because of their anatomy. Botulinum toxin injection can soften the glabellar ridge and decrease the appearance of aggressiveness and age. The glabella was the fourth most common area of concern in the survey by Jagdeo and colleagues.[3]

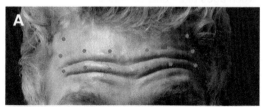
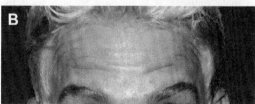

Fig. 1. A 52-year-old man before (*A*) and after (*B*) 36 units of abobotulinumtoxinA to the forehead (injection points are indicated by *blue dots*). Note the extra injection point in the frontotemporal hair line where the hairline recedes.

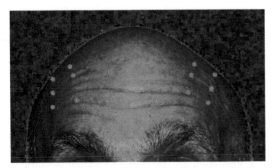

Fig. 2. In men with androgenetic alopecia, injection points should be extended into the frontal scalp.

Anatomy

Two corrugator supercilii, depressor supercilii, and a procerus contribute to glabellar lines. The corrugators originate from bone in the medial brow ridge and run along the orbital rim, ending more laterally and superiorly onto the frontalis muscle.[25] The corrugator supercilii extends farther laterally in men.[30] Vertical glabellar lines are formed by the corrugators. Anatomic studies have shown that the depressor supercilii originates from the frontal process of the maxilla, about 1 cm above the medial canthal tendon, traveling superiorly 4 to 5 mm before inserting into the dermis in the medial brow.[31] It acts as a brow depressor and may contribute to oblique glabellar lines. The procerus fibers originate from tendons in the inferior nasal bone, and interdigitate superiorly with the frontalis. Contraction of the procerus causes horizontal glabellar lines. In men, the glabella is wider and projects more anteriorly.[32] A study showed that men less than 65 years of age had more severe glabellar lines than women of the same age, although this was only statistically significant between ages of 21 and 28 years.[27]

Treatment goals

Unlike other areas of the face, total effacement of glabellar lines is often desired in male patients. Immobilizing the glabella alone can result in lifting of the lateral brow, because of unopposed action of the frontalis. Thus, when treating the glabella in male patients, it is prudent to also treat the forehead.

Dosing and injection technique

- The glabella is the only location where the dose of botulinum toxin was specifically studied in men. Carruthers and colleagues[19] injected the glabella of 80 male patients with 20, 40, 60, and 80 units of OBA. They found doses of 40 to 80 units were most effective and had the greatest duration compared with 20 units, without an increase in adverse events. A

previous study by the same investigators had shown that, in female patients, the glabellar complex should be treated with at least 20 units.[33] Carruthers and colleagues[33] recommend starting with 40 units in the male glabella.
- Brandt and colleagues[18] showed that, in 15 male and 90 female patients injected with 50 units of abobotulinumtoxinA (ABO), 67% of men, compared with 93% of women, obtained significant improvement of glabellar lines. The investigators concluded that men may need ABO doses greater than 50 units. Another trial supported the use of higher doses of ABO in men (60–80 units).[20]
- Two injections points are indicated for each corrugator, and 1 for the procerus (**Fig. 3**).
- When injecting the corrugators, stay at least 1 cm above the orbital rim to prevent diffusion into the levator palpebrae superioris. For the medial injection, identify the point of greatest muscle contraction. For the tail of the corrugator, Bloom and colleagues[34] recommend identifying the most lateral aspect of the corrugator (presence of dimpling) and placing the lateral injections just medial to this insertion point in the skin.
- Injections placed too superiorly in the mid glabella may also affect the medial frontalis, resulting in elevation of the lateral brow.[35]
- Avoid injecting the glabella alone in order to prevent elevation of the brow.

Periocular Skin

Like women, men develop periocular rhytides with age. Jagdeo and colleagues'[3] survey found that, along with the tear trough, the crow's feet is the facial area mostly likely to be treated in men.

Anatomy

The orbicularis oculi is a spherical muscle consisting of a lacrimal, palpebral, and orbital portion.[36] The orbital portion controls voluntary closure of the eyelids, creating dynamic lateral canthal lines. With time, these lines become static.[37] In men, the orbicularis oculi is broader and extends more laterally.[23,24] Men also tend to have predominantly a lower-fan pattern of lateral canthal lines, with greater recruitment of muscular elevators of the cheek.[38,39] In addition, the orbicularis oculi contributes to the palpebral aperture and infraorbital shelving and rhytides.[40]

Treatment goals

Lateral canthal lines in men can indicate maturity and contribute to attractiveness and the appearance of a positive disposition.[41] Thus, a goal for male patients may be just to soften these rhytides.

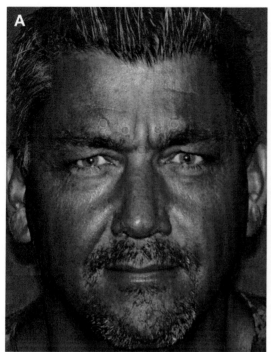
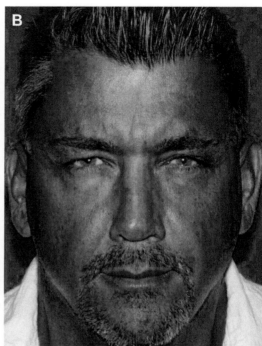

Fig. 3. A 49-year-old man before (*A*) and after (*B*) 30 units of onabotulinumtoxinA and 0.4 cm³ of hyaluronic acid filler to the glabella. It is important to maintain some level of movement in the glabellar complex in a man, for a more natural aesthetic.

Dosing and technique

- The FDA approved the use of OBA for lateral canthal lines in 2013. A phase 2 dose-ranging study showed that there was a greater responder rate with a total dose of 24 units rather than 6 or 12 units.[42] Of the 162 patients, only 11.1% were men, and no subgroup analysis was performed. The consensus recommendation for lateral canthal lines is 6 to 15 units per side.[28] For men, Flynn[43] recommends starting with 15 units of OBA per side.

- The most used technique for lateral canthal lines involves 3 injections (**Figs. 4** and **5**). One injection is placed at the level of the lateral canthus, 1 cm lateral to the orbital rim. The other 2 are placed 1.0 to 1.5 cm both superiorly and inferiorly, angled at 30° anterior to the first injection.[39] In patients with a lower-fan pattern of canthal lines, the other 2 injections can be placed anterior and inferior to the first injection. Some investigators add microdroplets (0.5 units) of toxin to the lateral inferior orbicularis oculi for lower fanning lines.[36,44] It is important to inject superficially, because the zygomaticus major may be as shallow as 0.41 cm deep to the orbicularis oculi.[45] Diffusion into the zygomaticus major or levator labii superioris can affect the smile. In addition, because men can have greater lateral fanning of the orbicularis oculi, a second row of injections is sometimes used.[36]

- Applying 1 to 2 units per side of OBA to the infraorbital eyelid (inferior orbicularis oculi muscle) can decrease lower eyelid rhytides and shelving, and increase the palpebral aperture. In a study of 15 women, this injection was shown to increase the palpebral aperture at rest by a mean of 0.5 mm, and by 1.8 mm if combined with treatment of lateral canthal lines.[40] The toxin is applied in the midpupillary line, 3 to 4 mm inferior to the lid margin. Before this injection, the physician should assess for lower scleral show and perform a snap test. Men have been found to have a greater degree of lower eyelid sagging, which increases the risk of adverse events with an inferior eyelid injection. In addition, the presence of lower eyelid and malar mound edema should be noted. Neurotoxin injection to the lower eyelid caused lower eyelid edema in 1% of patients in phase 3 trials.[46,47]

MIDFACE
Nose

In 2015, rhinoplasty was the most common procedure performed in men.[2] Because of the

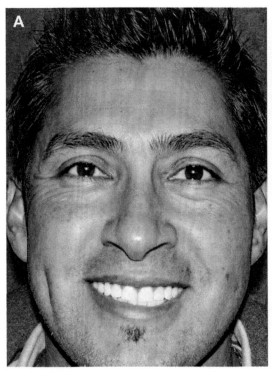
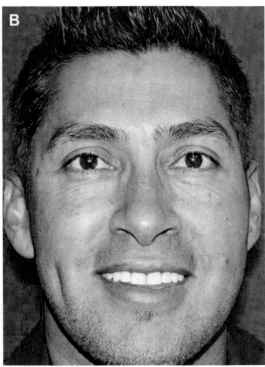

Fig. 4. A 42-year-old man before (*A*) and after (*B*) 12 units of onabotulinumtoxin A to each orbicularis oculi.

growing popularity of nonsurgical rhinoplasty, more men may seek hyaluronic acid filler and botulinum toxin to improve the appearance of their nose.

Anatomy

Various muscles contribute to the position and rhytides of the nose. The nasalis has a transverse and alar portion. The alar nasalis, present over the nasal ala, is involved in nasal flaring. Contraction of the transverse nasalis produces nasal oblique lines (also known as bunny lines). The

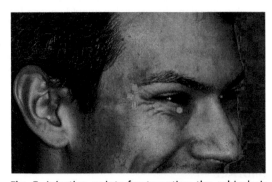

Fig. 5. Injection points for targeting the orbicularis oculi in a man with full-fan pattern of periocular rhytides, with a total of 12 units of onabotulinumtoxin A or 36 units of abobotulinumtoxinA per side.

depressor septi nasi causes the downward movement of the nasal tip during activities like speaking and smiling.[48] This muscle arises from the orbicularis oris and periosteum above the central and lateral incisors, then inserts onto the nasal septum or medial cura.[49] It is notable that the levator labii superioris alaeque nasi (LLSAN), procerus, orbicularis oculi, and zygomaticus major and minor also play a role in nasal movements and wrinkling.

Treatment goals

Patients who have had botulinum toxin to the upper face may notice that oblique nasal lines become more evident. The presence of oblique nasal lines has not been studied in men, but physicians should still assess for this possible area of concern (**Fig. 6**). Another concern for which men may seek treatment is nasal tip ptosis. As men age, the nasal tip descends. In patients in whom the ptosis worsens with muscle activity, botulinum to the depressor septi nasi may help. Excessive nasal tip elevation may feminize the patient, because the angle between the upper cutaneous lip and nasal tip tends to be 97° in men versus 104.9° in women.[50]

Dosing and injection technique

- Tamura and colleagues[51] treated 250 women with nasalis wrinkles with 3 units of

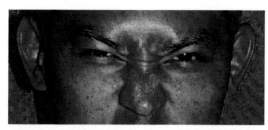

Fig. 6. This male patient recruits the nasalis when asked to frown. Thus, the nasalis should also be treated.

abobotulinumtoxinA to the transverse nasalis. They found that 60% had remaining rhytides around the ala and superior lateral nasal bridge. These patients required additional injection points to the LLSAN, nasal portion of the orbicularis oculi, and procerus, depending on where the wrinkles were observed. The consensus recommendation for bunny lines is a total of 4 to 8 units, or even as many as 10 units.[28]

- To target the depressor septi nasi, an injection is placed in the columella, just above its junction with the cutaneous upper lip. Redaelli[48] uses 1.5 units per side of the columella (total of 3 units). In that report, men made up 15 of 95 patients undergoing nonsurgical rhinoplasty with botulinum toxin and hyaluronic acid. The investigators did not comment on any gender-specific differences. The latest consensus recommends 2 to 6 units for the treatment of hyperdynamic tip ptosis.[29]
- To decrease nasal flaring, 1 to 2 units of toxin can be injected to the alar portion of each nasalis.[29]

Gingival Show

Excessive gingival show, otherwise known as a gummy smile, is defined as exposure of more than 2 mm of gingiva when smiling.[52] In cases in which it is caused by muscle hyperactivity, botulinum toxin can be used to decrease the show of the gum.

Anatomy

The LLSAN, levator labii superioris, levator anguli oris, zygomaticus major and minor, risorius, and depressor septi nasi all interact with the orbicularis oris to elevate and laterally retract the lip. The LLSAN originates from the frontal process of the maxilla, diving into 2 fascicles that attach to the skin and cartilage of the nasal ala and upper lip, dilating the nostrils and raising the upper lip.[53] The zygomaticus major and minor start at the superior lateral zygomatic bone, inserting at the modiolus and lateral upper lip, respectively.[54]

They move the upper lip upward and laterally, and work in smiling, chewing, and speaking. In a study of 16 patients, Mazzuco and colleagues[53] identified 4 types of gummy smiles. Anterior gummy smiles are characterized by gingival show primarily between the 2 canines, mainly caused by activity of the LLSAN. In a posterior gummy smile, gingival show is present posterior to the canines, and the zygomaticus major and minor are the main contributors. Mixed gummy smile has both anterior and posterior involvement, whereas asymmetric gummy smile has excessive exposure only on 1 side.

Treatment goals

It is thought that men have a lower incidence of excessive gingival show, because men overall have been found to have a predominantly low smile.[55] Polo[56] found that 76 of 8423 patients had gummy smile secondary to hyperfunctional lip levators. Of the 76, only 3 (3.95%) were male. Thus, gummy smile may be an uncommon complaint among male patients seeking cosmetic interventions.

Dosing and injection technique

- In 4 studies included in a systematic review by Nasr and colleagues,[52] doses ranging from 2 to 7.5 units per side were used. The consensus recommendation is 2 to 4 units per side.[29]
- To target the LLSAN, an injection can be placed 1 cm lateral to and below the nasal ala.[55]
- Injection of the zygomaticus major or minor muscles is a more advanced technique with higher risk of potential complications. Two injections are performed: the first on the nasolabial fold at the point of greatest muscle contraction and the second injection 2 cm lateral to the first point, at the level of the tragus.[55] In their study, Mazzuco and colleagues found a lower average improvement with posterior and mixed gummy smiles, which Nasr and colleagues[52] attributed to the LLSAN being crucial in the treatment of gummy smile. To target the LLSAN, levator labii superioris, and zygomaticus minor, Nasr and colleagues[52] recommended injecting at a point 1 cm lateral to the nasal ala and 3 cm above the lip line.[54]
- Side effects include smile asymmetry, lowering of the oral commissure, and difficulty with mouth functions.[54] Therefore, it is prudent to start with a lower unit dose and see the patient for follow-up.

LOWER FACE
Masseter

Hypertrophy of the masseter muscle can lead to a heavy lower face, square-appearing jawline, temporomandibular joint disorders, and bruxism.[57] Botulinum toxin injection can be used off-label to reduce masseter hypertrophy.

Anatomy

Xie and colleagues[58] used ultrasonography and cadaveric dissection to examine the anatomy of the masseter in 252 patients, 24 of whom were men. Another 220 patients underwent treatment with botulinum toxin, of whom 15 were men. Three muscle layers (superficial, middle, and deep) were identified, with the fibers arising from the zygomatic arch and inserting into the masseter tuberosity. With contraction of the muscle, the investigators classified 5 different bulging types: minimal, mono, double, triple, and excessive.

Treatment goals

Botulinum toxin to the masseter helps women achieve a narrow and rounded lower face. Compared with women, the male mandible is wider and has a more prominent flexure.[59] Thus, botulinum should be reserved for men whose masseter hypertrophy contributes to physical symptoms, imparts an overly masculine appearance to the mandibular angle, or causes facial asymmetry (**Fig. 7**).

Dosing and technique

- The dosing of botulinum for masseter injections should be based on muscle thickness, regardless of race, ethnicity, or gender.[34,60]

The latest consensus recommendation advises 15 to 40 units per masseter.[29]

- Xie and colleagues[58] used 20 to 25 units of OBA per masseter for muscles less than 10 mm thick, 25 to 30 units for masseters 10 to 13.9 mm thick, and 30 to 40 units for masseters more than 14 mm thick. Their injection technique was based on the number of bulges observed when clenching, performing 1 injection point per bulge. The maximum number of injections, even for excessive bulging, was 3. The greatest aesthetic effect and muscle atrophy occurred at 3 months postinjection. Patients who received higher doses had complication rates of 60%, compared with an overall complication rate of 9.1%. Asymmetric smile was the most common complication.

- Kim and colleagues[61] studied ABO in 1021 patients. Of these, 383 followed up longer than 3 months, of whom 28 were male. Doses ranged from 100 to 140 units of ABO per side based on muscle thickness. As seen in other studies, the maximum decrease in muscle volume occurred at 10 to 12 weeks, with a 31% mean reduction.

- Prior to starting, the safe zone of injection should be outlined (**Fig. 8**). A line drawn from the angle of the mouth to the lower implantation of the ear defines the superior border, and the mandible the inferior border.[34] With the patient clenching, the physician can assess the anterior and posterior borders of the masseter. Keeping injections 1 cm lateral to the anterior border of the masseter helps avoid diffusion into muscles of facial expression.[62] Although Xie and colleagues[58]

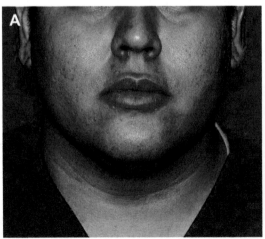
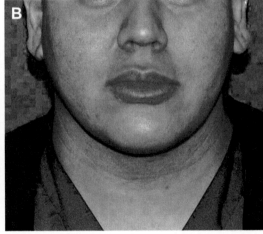

Fig. 7. A 26-year-old man before (*A*) and after (*B*) 30 units of onabotulinumtoxin A to each masseter to slim the face.

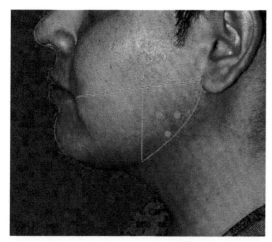

Fig. 8. The blue dotted line denotes the recommended borders of injection. A line can be drawn superiorly from the oral commissure to the lower insertion of the tragus, anteriorly by the anterior border of the masseter, and inferiorly and laterally by the angle of the mandible and posterior masseter. Injections should be kept 1 cm posterior to the anterior border to avoid diffusion into muscles of facial expression.

recommend basing the injections on the number of muscle bulges, most investigators prefer 3 injection points per masseter.[34,63]

- Masticatory weakness can develop at approximately 2 weeks postinjection, usually recovering by 3 weeks because of the likely compensation by other muscles of mastication.[63]

Perioral Lines

The orbicularis oris can be targeted with botulinum toxin to reduce perioral lines. However, this complaint may be uncommon in male patients. In cadaveric examinations, Paes and colleagues[64] found that male cadavers showed fewer and shallower perioral lines, likely because of a significantly higher concentration of sebaceous glands per hair follicle.

Anatomy

Similar to the orbicularis oculi, the orbicularis oris is a muscle that encircles the oral aperture. Its contraction leads to the formation of lines perpendicular to the vermillion border.

Treatment goals

In men who develop perioral lines, care must be taken to only decrease the activity of the orbicularis oris. Excessive immobilization can lead to difficulties with phonation, drinking, kissing, and playing musical instruments. It is best to start with lower doses and avoid treatment in musicians and singers.

Doing and technique

- Cohen and colleagues[65] performed a dose-ranging study using 7.5 or 12 units of OBA in 60 female subjects. Although efficacy measures were similar between the 2 doses, the 12-unit dose was associated with a greater number of adverse events. The consensus recommendation is a total of 1 to 5 units.[29]
- Dermal injections are placed along or up to 2 mm away from the vermillion border. The number of injection points should be based on the patient's specific rhytid pattern, but varies from 2 to 4 injections in the upper lip and 2 in the lower lip.[66] It is important to stay 1 cm medial to the oral commissures in order to avoid diffusion of the toxin into the modiolus.[67]

Chin

Loss of mandibular bone and subcutaneous fat, along with hyperactivity of the mentalis muscle, can lead to peau d'orange appearance of the chin and an accentuated horizontal chin crease.[68] A high riding mentalis may also alter the contour of the chin and position of the pogonion.[69]

Anatomy

The mentalis muscle everts the lower lip and elevates the soft tissues of the chin. It functions in the ability to pout. The 2 muscle bellies originate from the anterior mandible and insert superiorly into the soft tissue of the chin, connecting with the orbicularis oris and depressor labii inferioris (DLI).[70]

Treatment goals

Like the mandible, the chin is wider, and projects more anteriorly, in men.[71] For men who are concerned by a pebbled appearance or prominent chin crease, botulinum toxin can be used to the mentalis. Additionally, OBA injection to the mentalis has been shown to be able to shift the position of the pogonion inferiorly, and improve the contour of the chin on profile.[69]

Dosing and injection technique

- No dose-ranging studies have been performed for mentalis injections. Most investigators place a total of 4 to 10 units, either with 1 injection point in the midmandible where the 2 bellies insert or with 2 separate injections into each muscle belly, about 5 mm from the center of the chin.[72]
- In their trial on patients with a high riding, hyperactive mentalis, Hsu and colleagues injected 12 to 15 units of OBA in 2 to 3 unit aliquots. It is

important to keep injections medial and deep in order to avoid diffusion in to the DLI or depressor anguli oris (DAO).[67,70]

Depressor Anguli Oris

Loss of bone and soft tissue in the chin and medial cheek can cause decreased projection of the chin and downward displacement of the midface over the melomental folds, causing downward displacement of the oral commissures and marionette lines.[67]

Anatomy

The DAO is a fan-shaped muscle that originates at the mandible and inserts into the modiolus, interlacing with various adjacent muscles, including the DLI, mentalis, and plastysma.[73] The medial portion of the DAO lies deep to the DLI.[74] It functions in drawing the angle of the mouth inferiorly and laterally. DAO hyperactivity leads to melomental lines and downturning of the angle of the mouth.[74] Thus, botulinum toxin can allow the unopposed function of the primary mouth elevators, including the zygomaticus major and levator anguli oris.

Treatment goals

Because of the more sebaceous nature of male perioral skin, men may have a decreased incidence of marionette lines, although this has never been quantified. Tsukahara and colleagues[28] found that, in patients aged 65 to 75 years, women had significantly higher wrinkle scores in the corner of the mouth compared with men.

Dosing and injection technique

- Experts recommend 2 to 4 units per DAO.[29] A split-face study on 20 female subjects did not show a difference between 4 units (0.1 mL) of OBA and 10 units (0.1 mL) of ABO.[75] Both were equally effective in improving the appearance of the melomental folds at maximum contraction up to 16 weeks after the injection. No adverse events were reported.
- Avoiding affecting the DLI is of utmost importance when targeting the DAO. In order to minimize this risk, have the patient pull the corners of the mouth downward and laterally to identify the point of greatest contraction of the DAO (**Fig. 9**). This point should be at least 1 cm lateral to the oral commissure.[76] The injection is kept inferior to the mental foramen.[77]

Platysmal Bands

The platysma plays an integral part in the appearance of the neck and lower face. Botulinum toxin in

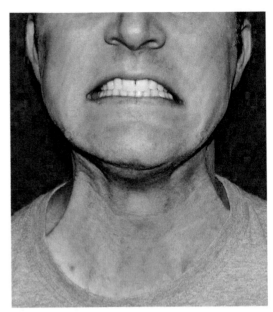

Fig. 9. The DAO can be identified by having patients show their bottom teeth. The injection point is commonly 1 cm posterior to a line extending from the nasolabial fold to the angle of the mandible. Classically 4 units of onabotulinumtoxin A or 12 units of abobotulinumtoxinA are placed into each DAO. This patient would benefit from more on his left than his right DAO.

the platysma can be used to rejuvenate these 2 areas.

Anatomy

The platysma is a broad and thin muscle that originates from the fascia of the upper chest and clavicle. It courses superiorly immediately below superficial neck fat, with fibers inserting into mandibular bone, DAO, DLI, modiolus, and the superficial aponeurotic system of the cheeks.[78,79] With contraction, the platysma pulls the clavicle upward and depresses the lower cheek and oral commissures. With time, hypertrophy of the platysma also leads to vertical platysmal bands, blunting of the cervicomental angle, and lowering of the corners of the mouth.[80]

Treatment goals

Although the male neck undergoes similar changes with aging as the female neck, the incidence of platysmal banding in men has not been specifically studied. Matarasso and colleagues[78] treated the platysmal banding of more than 1500 patients, of whom 16% were men. Appropriate patient selection is key in achieving successful results with botulinum toxin. Men with excessive skin laxity and fat deposits are better candidates for other procedures like liposuction, neck lift, or subsurface monopolar radiofrequency.

Dosing and injection technique

- For platysmal bands, space injections every 2 cm along a cord, using 2 to 4 units per injection site (**Fig. 10**). The needle is placed superficially, and it is helpful to hold the platysma between 2 fingers. High total doses and excessively deep injections can lead to weakness of the neck flexors, dysphagia, and dystonia.[76,81]
- There is a specific injection technique for patients in whom blunting of the mandibular border occurs with contraction of the platysma. In 2007, Levy[82] described the Nefertiti lift, named after an Egyptian queen. In addition to vertical injections into the platysmal bands, a horizontal line of 4 injections are placed along the superior platysma immediately below the mandibular bone.[83] These are spaced 1 to 2 cm apart, starting at least 1 cm posterior to where a line drawn from the nasolabial fold meets the mandible; this avoids the DLI.[84]
- Clinicians should not exceed a total of 50 units per injection session to avoid complications.[84] Matarasso and colleagues[78] used between 50 and 100 units of OBA, with 1 injector using up to 250 units. Of the patients treated, 1% developed neck weakness while lifting their heads, and 1 patient reported dysphagia for 14 days.

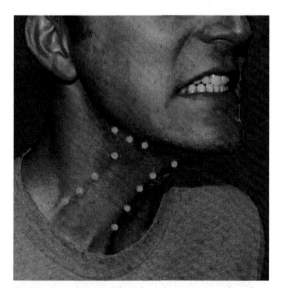

Fig. 10. For platysmal bands, injections are placed superficially, spaced every 2 cm along each cord, with 2 units of onabotulinumtoxin A or 6 units of abobotulinumtoxinA into each injection point. The superior row of injection points along the mandible receives 4 units of onabotulinumtoxin A or 12 units of abobotulinumtoxinA into each injection point to provide greater jawline definition.

SUMMARY

Male patients require a gender-specific approach to the injection of botulinum toxin. This article reviews how men have unique goals, expectations, and anatomy, and require differing doses and techniques. These recommendations are based on the available body of evidence and expert recommendations. However, this literature remains sparse, and many questions remain regarding sex differences in the use of botulinum toxin. These questions include whether there are biological variances in the binding and diffusion of botulinum toxin, and whether male patients require different dosing in areas other than the upper face. With continued interest and research in male aesthetics, physicians will continue to improve their care of male patients.

REFERENCES

1. 2016 National Plastic Surgery Statistics. American Society of Plastic Surgeons Web site. Available at: https://d2wirczt3b6wjm.cloudfront.net/News/Statistics/2016/2016-plastic-surgery-statistics-report.pdf. Accessed March 25, 2017.
2. 2015 Plastic Surgery Statistics Report. American Society of Plastic Surgeons Web site. Available at: https://d2wirczt3b6wjm.cloudfront.net/News/Statistics/2015/cosmetic-procedures-men-2015.pdf. Accessed March 25, 2017.
3. Jagdeo J, Keaney T, Narurkar V, et al. Facial treatment preferences among aesthetically oriented men. Dermatol Surg 2016;42(10):1155–63.
4. 2004 Membership Survey: Trends in facial plastic surgery, March 2005. American Academy of Facial Plastic and Reconstructive Surgery Web site. Available at: http://www.aafprs.org. Accessed February 2, 2017.
5. Carruthers A, Gallagher C, Darmody S. Evolution of facial aesthetic treatment over 5 or more years: an international, retrospective, cross-sectional analysis of continuous onabotulinumtoxinA treatment. J Am Acad Dermatol 2014;70:AB17.
6. Baker DC, Stefani WA, Chiu ES. Reducing the incidence of hematoma requiring surgical evacuation following male rhytidectomy: a 30-year review of 985 cases. Plast Reconstr Surg 2005;116:1973–85.
7. Moretti G, Ellis RA, Mescon H. Vascular patterns in the skin of the face. J Invest Dermatol 1959;33:103–12.
8. Mayrovitz HN, Regan MB. Gender differences in facial skin blood perfusion during basal and heated conditions determined by laser Doppler flowmetry. Microvasc Res 1993;45:211–8.
9. Montagna W, Ellis RA. Histology and cytochemistry of human skin. XIII. The blood supply of the hair follicle. J Natl Cancer Inst 1957;19:451–63.

10. Alam M, Geisler A, Sadhwani D, et al. Effect of needle size on pain perception in patients treated with botulinum toxin type A injections: a randomized clinical trial. JAMA Dermatol 2015;151(11):1194–9.

11. Lacy DB, Tepp W, Cohen AC, et al. Crystal structure of botulinum neurotoxin type A and implications for toxicity. Nat Struct Biol 1998;5:898–902.

12. Schiavo G, Matteoli M, Montecucco C. Neurotoxins affecting neuroexocytosis. Physiol Rev 2000;80: 717–66.

13. Hexsel D, Hexsel C, Siega C, et al. Fields of effects of 2 commercial preparations of botulinum toxin type A at equal labeled unit doses: a double-blind randomized trial. JAMA Dermatol 2013;149:1386–91.

14. Ranoux D, Gury C, Fondarai J, et al. Respective potencies of onabotulinum A (Botox, Allergan Inc., Irvine CA, USA) and Dysport: a double blind, randomized, crossover study in cervical dystonia. J Neurol Neurosurg Psychiatry 2002; 72:459–62.

15. Hexsel D, Brum C, do Prado DZ, et al. Field effect of two commercial preparations of botulinum toxin type A: a prospective, double-blind, randomized clinical trial. J Am Acad Dermatol 2012;67(2):226–32.

16. Karsai S, Adrian R, Hammes S, et al. A randomized double-blind study of the effect of Botox and Dysport/Reloxin on forehead wrinkles and electromyographic activity. Arch Dermatol 2007;143(11): 1447–9.

17. Karsai S, Raulin C. Current evidence on the unit equivalence of different botulinum neurotoxin A formulations and recommendations for clinical practice in dermatology. Dermatol Surg 2009;35(1):1–8.

18. Brandt F, Swanson N, Baumann L, et al. Randomized, placebo-controlled study of a new botulinum toxin type a for treatment of glabellar lines: efficacy and safety. Dermatol Surg 2009;35(12):1893–901.

19. Carruthers A, Carruthers J. Prospective, double-blind, randomized, parallel-group, dose-ranging study of botulinum toxin type A in men with glabellar rhytids. Dermatol Surg 2005;31(10):1297–303.

20. Kane MA, Brandt F, Rohrich RJ, et al. Evaluation of variable-dose treatment with a new U.S. botulinum toxin type A (Dysport) for correction of moderate to severe glabellar lines: results from a phase III, randomized, double-blind, placebo-controlled study. Plast Reconstr Surg 2009;124(5):1619–29.

21. Janssen I, Heymsfield SB, Wang ZM, et al. Skeletal muscle mass and distribution in 468 men and women aged 18-88 yr. J Appl Physiol (1985) 2000; 89(1):81–8.

22. Bhasin S, Storer TW, Berman N, et al. The effects of supraphysiologic doses of testosterone on muscle size and strength in normal men. N Engl J Med 1996;335(1):1–7.

23. Weeden JC, Trotman CA, Faraway JJ. Three dimensional analysis of facial movement in normal adults: influence of sex and facial shape. Angle Orthod 2001;71:132–40.

24. Houstis O, Kiliaridis S. Gender and age differences in facial expressions. Eur J Orthod 2009;31:459–66.

25. Lorenc ZP, Smith S, Nestor M, et al. Understanding the functional anatomy of the frontalis and glabellar complex for optimal aesthetic botulinum toxin type A therapy. Aesthetic Plast Surg 2013;37(5): 975–83.

26. Whitaker LA, Morales L, Farkas LG. Aesthetic surgery of the supraorbital ridge and forehead structures. Plast Reconstr Surg 1986;78(1):23–32.

27. Goldstein SM, Katowitz JA. The male eyebrow: a topographic anatomic analysis. Ophthal Plast Reconstr Surg 2005;21:285–91.

28. Tsukahara K, Hotta M, Osanai O, et al. Gender dependent differences in degree of facial wrinkles. Skin Res Technol 2013;19(1):65–71.

29. Sundaram H, Liew S, Signorini M, et al. Global aesthetics consensus: botulinum toxin type A evidence-based review, emerging concepts, and consensus recommendations for aesthetic use, including updates on complications. Plast Reconstr Surg 2016; 137(3):518e–29e.

30. Macdonald MR, Spiegel JH, Raven RB, et al. An anatomical approach to glabellar rhytids. Arch Otolaryngol Head Neck Surg 1998;124:1315–20.

31. Cook BE Jr, Lucarelli MJ, Lemke BN. Depressor supercilii muscle: anatomy, histology, and cosmetic implications. Ophthal Plast Reconstr Surg 2001; 17(6):404–11.

32. Russell MD. The supraorbital torus: a most remarkable peculiarity. Curr Anthropol 1985;26:337–60.

33. Carruthers A, Carruthers J, Said S. Dose-ranging study of botulinum toxin type A in the treatment of glabellar rhytids in females. Dermatol Surg 2005; 31(4):414–22 [discussion: 422].

34. Bloom JD, Green JB, Bowe W, et al. Cosmetic use of abobotulinumtoxinA in men: considerations regarding anatomical differences and product characteristics. J Drugs Dermatol 2016;15(9):1056–62.

35. Ascher B, Zakine B, Kestemont P, et al. A multicenter, randomized, double-blind, placebo-controlled study of efficacy and safety of 3 doses of botulinum toxin A in the treatment of glabellar lines. J Am Acad Dermatol 2004;51:223–33.

36. Kim DW, Cundiff J, Toriumi DM. Botulinum toxin A for the treatment of lateral periorbital rhytids. Facial Plast Surg Clin North Am 2003;11(4):445–51.

37. Lemperle G, Holmes RE, Cohen SR, et al. A classification of facial wrinkles. Plast Reconstr Surg 2001;108(6):1735–50.

38. Kane MAC, Cox SE, Jones D, et al. Heterogeneity of crow's feet lines patterns in clinical trial subjects. Dermatol Surg 2015;41(4):447–56.

39. Carruthers A, Bruce S, Cox SE, et al. OnabotulinumtoxinA for treatment of moderate to severe

crow's feet lines: a review. Aesthet Surg J 2016; 36(5):591–7.

40. Flynn TC, Carruthers JA, Carruthers JA. Botulinum-A toxin treatment of the lower eyelid improves infraorbital rhytides and widens the eye. Dermatol Surg 2001;27(8):703–8.

41. Dayan SH, Ashourian N. Considerations for achieving a natural face in cosmetic procedures. JAMA Facial Plast Surg 2015;17(6):395.

42. Lowe NJ, Ascher B, Heckmann M, et al. Double-blind, randomized, placebo-controlled, dose-response study of the safety and efficacy of botulinum toxin type A in subjects with crow's feet. Dermatol Surg 2005;31(3):257–62.

43. Flynn TC. Botox in men. Dermatol Ther 2007;20(6): 407–13.

44. Monheit G. Neurotoxins: current concepts in cosmetic use on the face and neck–upper face (glabella, forehead, and crow's feet). Plast Reconstr Surg 2015;136(5 Suppl):72S–5S.

45. Spiegel JH, DeRosa J. The anatomical relationship between the orbicularis oculi muscle and the levator labii superioris and zygomaticus muscle complexes. Plast Reconstr Surg 2005;116(7):1937–42 [discussion: 1943–4].

46. Carruthers A, Bruce S, de Coninck A, et al. Efficacy and safety of onabotulinumtoxinA for the treatment of crow's feet lines: a multicenter, randomized, controlled trial. Dermatol Surg 2014;40(11):1181–90.

47. Moers-Carpi M, Carruthers J, Fagien S, et al. Efficacy and safety of onabotulinumtoxinA for treating crow's feet lines alone or in combination with glabellar lines: a multicenter, randomized, controlled trial. Dermatol Surg 2015;41(1):102–12.

48. Redaelli A. Medical rhinoplasty with hyaluronic acid and botulinum toxin A: a very simple and quite effective technique. J Cosmet Dermatol 2008;7(3): 210–20.

49. Rohrich RJ, Huynh B, Muzaffar AR, et al. Importance of the depressor septi nasi muscle in rhinoplasty: anatomic study and clinical application. Plast Reconstr Surg 2000;105(1):376–83 [discussion: 384–8].

50. Sinno HH, Markarian MK, Ibrahim AM, et al. The ideal nasolabial angle in rhinoplasty: a preference analysis of the general population. Plast Reconstr Surg 2014;134(2):201–10.

51. Tamura BM, Odo MY, Chang B, et al. Treatment of nasal wrinkles with botulinum toxin. Dermatol Surg 2005;31(3):271–5.

52. Nasr MW, Jabbour SF, Sidaoui JA, et al. Botulinum toxin for the treatment of excessive gingival display: a systematic review. Aesthet Surg J 2016;36(1):82–8.

53. Mazzuco R, Hexsel D. Gummy smile and botulinum toxin: a new approach based on the gingival exposure area. J Am Acad Dermatol 2010;63(6): 1042–51.

54. Shim KS, Hu KS, Kwak HH, et al. An anatomical study of the insertion of the zygomaticus major muscle in humans focused on the muscle arrangement at the corner of the mouth. Plast Reconstr Surg 2008;121:466–73.

55. Tjan AH, Miller GD, The JG. Some esthetic factors in a smile. J Prosthet Dent 1984;51:24–8.

56. Polo M. Botulinum toxin type A (Botox) for the neuromuscular correction of excessive gingival display on smiling (gummy smile). Am J Orthod Dentofacial Orthop 2008;133(2):195–203.

57. Long H, Liao Z, Wang Y, et al. Efficacy of botulinum toxins on bruxism: an evidence-based review. Int Dent J 2012;62(1):1–5.

58. Xie Y, Zhou J, Li H, et al. Classification of masseter hypertrophy for tailored botulinum toxin type a treatment. Plast Reconstr Surg 2014;134(2):209e–18e.

59. Garvin HM, Ruff CB. Sexual dimorphism in skeletal browridge and chin morphologies determined using a new quantitative method. Am J Phys Anthropol 2012;147(4):661–70.

60. Liew S, Dart A. Nonsurgical reshaping of the lower face. Aesthet Surg J 2008;28(3):251–7.

61. Kim NH, Chung JH, Park RH, et al. The use of botulinum toxin type A in aesthetic mandibular contouring. Plast Reconstr Surg 2005;115(3):919–30.

62. Bae JH, Choi DY, Lee JG, et al. The risorius muscle: anatomic considerations with reference to botulinum neurotoxin injection for masseteric hypertrophy. Dermatol Surg 2014;40(12):1334–9.

63. Klein FH, Brenner FM, Sato MS, et al. Lower facial remodeling with botulinum toxin type A for the treatment of masseter hypertrophy. An Bras Dermatol 2014;89(6):878–84.

64. Paes EC, Teepen HJ, Koop WA, et al. Perioral wrinkles: histologic differences between men and women. Aesthet Surg J 2009;29:467–72.

65. Cohen JL, Dayan SH, Cox SE, et al. OnabotulinumtoxinA dose-ranging study for hyperdynamic perioral lines. Dermatol Surg 2012;38(9):1497–505.

66. Semchyshyn N, Sengelmann RD. Botulinum toxin A treatment of perioral rhytides. Dermatol Surg 2003; 29:490–5.

67. Wu DC, Fabi SG, Goldman MP. Neurotoxins: current concepts in cosmetic use on the face and neck–lower face. Plast Reconstr Surg 2015;136(5 Suppl): 76S–9S.

68. Carruthers JD, Glogau RG, Blitzer A. Advances in facial rejuvenation: botulinum toxin type A, hyaluronic acid dermal fillers, and combination therapies – consensus recommendations. Plast Reconstr Surg 2008;121:5S–30S.

69. Hsu AK, Frankel AS. Modification of Chin Projection and Aesthetics With OnabotulinumtoxinA Injection. JAMA Facial Plast Surg 2017.

70. Hur MS, Kim HJ, Choi BY, et al. Morphology of the mentalis muscle and its relationship with the

orbicularis oris and incisivus labii inferioris muscles. J Craniofac Surg 2013;24:602–4.

71. Thayer ZM, Dobson SD. Sexual dimorphism in chin shape: implications for adaptive hypotheses. Am J Phys Anthropol 2010;143:417–25.

72. Raspaldo H, Niforos FR, Gassia V, et al. Lower-face and neck antiaging treatment and prevention using onabotulinumtoxin A: the 2010 multidisciplinary French consensus–part 2. J Cosmet Dermatol 2011;10(2):131–49.

73. Choi YJ, Kim JS, Gil YC, et al. Anatomical considerations regarding the location and boundary of the depressor anguli oris muscle with reference to botulinum toxin injection. Plast Reconstr Surg 2014; 134(5):917–21.

74. Hur MS, Kim HJ, Lee KS. An anatomic study of the medial fibers of depressor anguli oris muscle passing deep to the depressor labii inferioris muscle. J Craniofac Surg 2014;25(2):614–6.

75. Fabi SG, Massaki AN, Guiha I, et al. Randomized split-face study to assess the efficacy and safety of abobotulinumtoxina versus onabotulinumtoxina in the treatment of melomental folds (depressor anguli oris). Dermatol Surg 2015;41(11):1323–5.

76. Carruthers J, Carruthers A. Aesthetic botulinum A toxin in the mid and lower face and neck. Dermatol Surg 2003;29:468–76.

77. Hur MS, Hu KS, Cho JY, et al. Topography and location of the depressor anguli oris muscle with a reference to the mental foramen. Surg Radiol Anat 2008; 30:403–7.

78. Matarasso A, Matarasso SL, Brandt FS, et al. Botulinum A exotoxin for the management of platysma bands. Plast Reconstr Surg 1999;103(2):645–52 [discussion: 653–5].

79. Hoefflin SM. Anatomy of the platysma and lip depressor muscles. A simplified mnemonic approach. Dermatol Surg 1998;24(11):1225–31.

80. Brandt FS, Boker A. Botulinum toxin for the treatment of neck lines and neck bands. Dermatol Clin 2004; 22:159–66.

81. Carruthers J, Carruthers A. Practical cosmetic Botox techniques. J Cutan Med Surg 1999; 3(Suppl 4):S4–9.

82. Levy PM. The 'Nefertiti lift': a new technique for specific re-contouring of the jawline. J Cosmet Laser Ther 2007;9:249–52.

83. de Almeida AR, Romiti A, Carruthers JD. The facial platysma and its underappreciated role in lower face dynamics and contour. Dermatol Surg 2017; 43(8):1042–9.

84. Levy PM. Neurotoxins: current concepts in cosmetic use on the face and neck–jawline contouring/platysma bands/necklace lines. Plast Reconstr Surg 2015;136(5 Suppl):80S–3S.

Volumetric Structural Rejuvenation for the Male Face

Neil S. Sadick, MD[a,b],*

KEYWORDS

- Toxins • Volumetric structural rejuvenation • Facial aging • Matrix degradation

KEY POINTS

- Among the most popular noninvasive cosmetic treatments men seek today are fillers and toxins.
- Volumetric structural rejuvenation can be applied to both genders, but particularly when customizing this approach to men, it is of essence to know the key anatomic differences between the 2 sexes to avoid potential feminization.
- Volumetric structural rejuvenation is a term used to describe the technique of naturally restoring the face structure.

INTRODUCTION

Among the most popular non-invasive cosmetic treatments men seek today are fillers and toxins. Aside from safe and effective, these treatments are quick, require no downtime; the immediately visible results can boost a man's self-esteem, confidence, youthfulness, and sense of competitiveness in the personal and professional realms of the world. Clinically, the approach to using these agents increasingly and fundamentally has changed from ironing out the skin to remove wrinkles and lines to a highly-sophisticated restructuring of the 3-dimensional face. This new strategy, applied to and individualized according to each patient's goals and needs, relies on intimate knowledge of facial anatomy and the pathophysiology of aging. Volumetric structural rejuvenation (VSR) is a term coined by the author to describe the technique of naturally restoring the face structure, and also hints at the philosophy behind it: rejuvenating the face for natural aesthetic outcomes.[1] VSR can be applied to both genders, but particularly when customizing this approach to men, it is of essence to know the key anatomic differences between the 2 sexes to avoid potential feminization.

PATHOPHYSIOLOGY OF AGING IN MEN

Facial aging is characterized by a myriad of changes that affect the skin, musculature, adipose and skeletal compartments. These include photoaging, wrinkles, ptosis, and volume changes, that together via a complex interplay manifest to an aged face appearance (**Fig. 1**).

Skin

Men have thicker dermis, but matrix degradation during skin aging due to intrinsic (genetics) and extrinsic factors (UV radiation, smoking) generates reactive oxygen species (ROS), leading to the appearance of increased skin laxity or prominent folds around the nasolabial region, periorbital region, and jowl.[2] Moreover, studies have shown that men are more likely engage in lifestyle habits

---

Disclosure Statement: N. Sadick has nothing he wishes to disclose.
[a] Department of Dermatology, Weill Cornell Medicine, 1305 York Avenue, 70th Street, 9th floor, New York, NY 10021, USA; [b] Department of Dermatology, University of Buffalo, 1001 Main Street, Room 5154, Buffalo, NY 14203, USA
* Sadick Dermatology, 911 Park Avenue, Suite 1A, New York, NY 10075.
E-mail address: nssderm@sadickdermatology.com

Dermatol Clin 36 (2018) 43–48
https://doi.org/10.1016/j.det.2017.09.006
0733-8635/18/© 2017 Elsevier Inc. All rights reserved.

Younger

Older

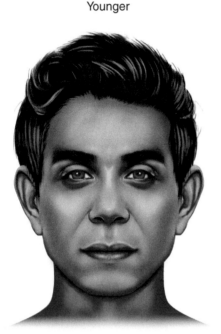
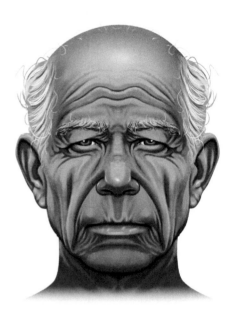

Fig. 1. Youthful and aged male face.

(smoking, less than rigorous use of sunscreen) that aggravate skin aging.[3]

Fat

As the face ages, redistribution and descent of facial fat pads contribute to the signature look of being older[4] (see **Fig. 1**). Facial fat has been shown to be partitioned between superficial and deep fat, organized in discrete anatomic compartments. The deep fat acts as the structural foundation over which subcutaneous fat lies. Age-related depletion of these fat pads results and loss of their even distribution, leading to predictable change in the appearance of the aged face, where sagging and hollowness persist. Specific areas that contribute to this look include diminishing of the cheek projection, atrophy in the periorbital, forehead, temporal, and perioral areas, leading to sagging due to the relative excess of remaining skin.[5] Although both genders sustain similar age-related changes of the adipose tissues, because men have less subcutaneous adipose tissue, they develop more prominent deep wrinkles rather than the fine lines observed in women.[6]

Bone

Craniofacial remodeling caused by aging also substantially impacts facial features and overall male aesthetics. Consistent age-related skeletal changes in both genders include an increase in mandibular angle that may cause blunting or loss of definition of the lower border of the face and an increase in the pyriform aperture that can lead to an appearance of nose elongation.[7] Midfacial bone loss may exacerbate the nasolabial fold appearance.[8] In men, as the forehead is oblique, the glabella and frontonasal suture are more pronounced, the supraorbital rim is prominent and the mandibular is angular, bone resorption leads to a general look of droopiness in the upper midface areas, and loss of the signature feature of male attractiveness, the strong square chin.[9]

OVERVIEW OF THE VOLUMETRIC STRUCTURAL REJUVENATION TECHNIQUE

The VSR methodology is designed with the aim to structurally reconstruct the face and replete tissues (fat, skeleton, skin) that have been resorbed because of the aging process. VSR is based on the bimodal trivector approach, where filler injections are placed at 3 sites (see **Fig. 1**) and at 2 levels: a deep dermal/supraosteal level and a subcutaneous level.[1]

The first step when performing the bimodal trivector approach involves supraperiosteal injections in the upper, middle, and lower face, thus reintroducing to the face a structural platform by mimicking the volume lost in the supportive temporal, preaurical, lateral cheek, midcheek, and mandibular fat pads and by addressing musculoskeletal atrophy. Three injection points are strategically selected and injected (**Fig. 2**), to not only address specific age-related indications, but to also minimize patient discomfort.

The first injection access point is in the temporal fossa to address forehead atrophy and brow ptosis, followed by the midface to treat the tear-trough, perinasal, and malar fat pad areas, and finally in the jaw line to address the mandibular angle, maxilla, and marionette lines.[10] The amount of product used varies from 1 to 2 mL in the temple, 2 to 4-mL in the cheek, and 1 to 2-mL perioral area. In men, so as to avoid feminization, reduced amounts of filler are advised in the temple and cheek area, whereas in the perioral area a minimum amount is required. All injections are depot injections and when fanning from an injection point, it is important to avoid multiple deposits at the apex of the fan.[11] Augmentation of the temple area should use the periosteal, depot injection technique, and although injections around the orbits also use periosteal placement, they should not be attempted without sufficient training. The malar augmentation technique involves placement immediately below the zygomatic bony prominence, directly above the periosteum over the maxillary bone, with linear threading and retrograde deposition of product.

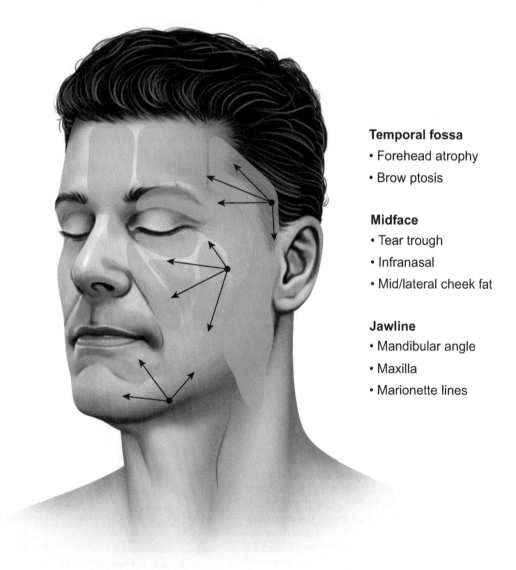

Temporal fossa
- Forehead atrophy
- Brow ptosis

Midface
- Tear trough
- Infranasal
- Mid/lateral cheek fat

Jawline
- Mandibular angle
- Maxilla
- Marionette lines

Fig. 2. The trivector sites of injection during the bimodal trivector approach.

Following injections at the trivector sites and the establishment of a structural platform, areas of superficial lipoatrophy are treated via customized deep dermal/subcutaneous injections. The goal of these injections is to individualize the volumetric filling in accordance with patient preferences and desired outcomes. These injections at the second step during the bimodal technique should be performed using a 27-gauge needle (0.5, 1.0, or 1.5 in) at a 30° to 40° entry angle and 0.1 to 0.2 mL aliquots of filler.[12]

VOLUMETRIC STRUCTURAL REJUVENATION IN MEN

When performing VSR in men, some important points need to be agreed upon during the consultation process. Depending on the gravity of the facial aging manifestations and the patient's goals, the amount of filler and choice of agent are decided. Hands-on examination including tissue palpation is used to identify anatomic landmarks such as the fat pads, bone and muscle structures, and the folds, wrinkles and creases that need to be treated. Aside from reversing the signs of aging, fillers can also be used to augment masculine facial features, notably by adding definition in the chin and jaw area or in the upper face to enhance the male forehead prominence by injecting the material into the bony sulcus over the eyebrows.[13] However, caution needs to be exercised when injecting in these areas as overcorrection, especially by administering too much volume medially or laterally, can result in a feminine appearance. Another gender-related anatomic difference that should be considered when performing filler injections in men is that men have a greater density of superficial blood vessels in the face than women, which makes men more prone to develop bruising. This adverse effect can be circumvented using a cannula instead of a needle, which has been shown to minimize vascular injury and subsequent bruising.[14]

VOLUMETRIC FILLERS FOR VOLUMETRIC STRUCTURAL REJUVENATION IN MEN

There is a myriad of filler options available for physicians to successfully apply the VSR technique in men: hyaluronic acid (HA), calcium hydroxylapatite (CaHA), poly-L-lactic acid (PLLA), and polymethyl methacrylate (PMMA). All of these products can provide panfacial augmentation in the trivector sites of lipoatrophy, but can also be utilized for customizing individual results, depending on the patient's goals and desires. Typically, men do not want a series of treatments and prefer to see

immediate, durable volumizing results. In this sense, new-generation high molecule HA fillers are ideal, as they can volumize the face and last up to 2 years.[15] In contrast to some of the other fillers (PLLA, PMMA), HA does not have as strong biostimulatory activity; thus the amount of filler used should be estimated according to the patient's face, all while avoiding overcorrection that can feminize it.

Juvéderm Voluma (Allergan, California), a 20 mg/mL HA dermal filler using the Vycross cross-linking technology, was approved by the US Food and Drug Administration (FDA) in 2013 as the first dermal filler for treatment of age-related volume loss in the midface. Because of its high HA concentration and high G prime, which translates into lift capacity and cohesivity, Voluma can successfully provide vertical lift adding structure, form, and volume.[16] When performing VSR, Voluma can be used for the supraosteal injections, whereas another HA filler from the Juvéderm series, Volbella (approved by the FDA in 2016), with its lower concentration at 15 mg/mL, a lower G prime, and cohesivity can be used for superficial injections to reduce lines, and more subtle depressions. Restylane Defyne by Galderma, which also recently won FDA approval, uses a cross-linking technology called XpresHAn technology, which creates a smooth flexible gel, for natural durable panfacial augmentation results. This filler is popular with men who show a strong preference for discreet results.

CaHa (Radiesse, Merz) is another filler that can be used for applying the VSR technique in men. As the CaHa particles are larger, and men's skin is thicker, deep supraosteal CaHa injections can restore the depleted adipose structural framework, while superficial injections for customized refining can be used with either CaHa or another

A   **B**

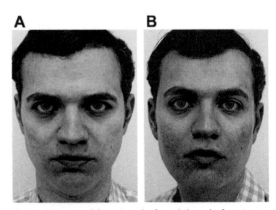

Fig. 3. 30-year-old patient before (A) and after 1 year (B) of Sculptra injections in the midface, mandible, and temple area.

A   B

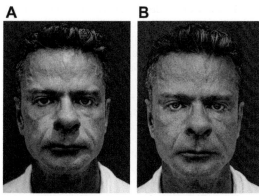

Fig. 4. 60-year-old patient before (*A*) and after 2 years (*B*) of Bellafill injections in the midface, mandible, and temple area.

filler type such as a low-viscosity HA filler.[17] Often a different kind of filler is chosen for the subcutaneous injections, as common side effects of CaHa include nodules, particularly in sites of facial dynamic movement.

Injectable PLLA (Sculptra, Galderma) is also commonly used for VSR in men (**Fig. 3**). Although it is not well suited to address fine rhytides or lip volume, it has other properties such as biostimulatory activity that can improve skin quality due to enhanced collagen/elastin remodeling.[18,19] Thus, using PLLA in men with poor skin quality can not only address sites of lipoatrophy, but also provide additional skin rejuvenation. It is important when using PLLA to under-correct as the filler continues to correct and volumize the face in the months following the injections.

Finally, PMMA (Bellafill, Suneva) is a permanent FDA-approved filler for the treatment of nasolabial folds.[20] Off-label use of PMMA has been shown for several other areas, and there has been success in its use for panfacial augmentation. PMMA can be appealing to men, because it is the only permanent filler that provides immediate volumization (**Fig. 4**).

SUMMARY

VSR is a comprehensive method that addresses facial aging by considering the entire face, its structural framework, and specific patient goals. For men, it can satisfy their needs for both reversing the signs of aging but also age prophylaxis and accentuation of specific male features, without surgery, downtime, or excess costs. It is advisable the VSR methodology is incorporated in a holistic program that involves tending to the epidermis with the use of sunscreens and topicals containing growth factors/antioxidants, and the

dermis with the stimulation of collagen/elastin remodeling via energy-based technologies (radiofrequency, laser, light, ultrasound). The combination of volumetric injectable fillers with neurotoxins, topical care, and energy-based devices is a noninvasive way that may help forestall the facial aging process and provide more natural results than are possible with any of these techniques alone. For men, as discreet, speedy, pain-free, low-maintenance options are of the essence, it is important for physicians to be able to design a same-day combination protocol of VSR together with other treatments to exceed patient expectations and ensure the highest level of satisfaction. Together with high-level evidence clinical studies describing protocols and results in male-only subjects, this growing patient demographic will slowly but surely be commonly and openly entering and treated in the clinic.

REFERENCES

1. Sadick NS, Manhas-Bhutani S, Krueger N. A novel approach to structural facial volume replacement. Aesthetic Plast Surg 2013;37(2):266–76.
2. Hamra ST. The role of orbital fat preservation in facial aesthetic surgery. A new concept. Clin Plast Surg 1996;23(1):17–28.
3. Antonov D, Hollunder M, Schliemann S, et al. Ultraviolet exposure and protection behavior in the general population: a structured interview survey. Dermatology 2016;232(1):11–6.
4. Sadick NS, Dorizas AS, Krueger N, et al. The facial adipose system: its role in facial aging and approaches to volume restoration. Dermatol Surg 2015;41(Suppl 1):S333–9.
5. Donofrio LM. Fat distribution: a morphologic study of the aging face. Dermatol Surg 2000;26(12):1107–12.
6. Sjöström L, Smith U, Krotkiewski M, et al. Cellularity in different regions of adipose tissue in young men and women. Metabolism 1972;21(12):1143–53.
7. Shaw RB Jr, Katzel EB, Koltz PF, et al. Aging of the mandible and its aesthetic implications. Plast Reconstr Surg 2010;125(1):332–42.
8. Lewis CD, Perry JD. A paradigm shift: volume augmentation or 'inflation' to obtain optimal cosmetic results. Curr Opin Ophthalmol 2009;20(5):389–94.
9. Farhadian JA, Bloom BS, Brauer JA. Male aesthetics: a review of facial anatomy and pertinent clinical implications. J Drugs Dermatol 2015;14(9):1029–34.
10. Rohrich RJ, Pessa JE. The fat compartments of the face: anatomy and clinical implications for cosmetic surgery. Plast Reconstr Surg 2007;119(7):2219–27 [discussion: 2228–31].
11. Fitzgerald R, Vleggaar D. Facial volume restoration of the aging face with poly-l-lactic acid. Dermatol Ther 2011;24(1):2–27.

12. Fitzgerald R, Vleggaar D. Using poly-L-lactic acid (PLLA) to mimic volume in multiple tissue layers. J Drugs Dermatol 2009;8(10 Suppl):s5–14.

13. de Maio M. Ethnic and gender considerations in the use of facial injectables: male patients. Plast Reconstr Surg 2015;136(5 Suppl):40S–3S.

14. van Loghem JA, Humzah D, Kerscher M. Cannula versus sharp needle for placement of soft tissue fillers: an observational cadaver study. Aesthet Surg J 2016. [Epub ahead of print].

15. Scherer MA. Specific aspects of a combined approach to male face correction: botulinum toxin A and volumetric fillers. J Cosmet Dermatol 2016; 15(4):566–74.

16. Goodman GJ, Swift A, Remington BK. Current concepts in the use of Voluma, Volift, and Volbella. Plast Reconstr Surg 2015;136(5 Suppl):139S–48S.

17. Sadick NS, Katz BE, Roy D. A multicenter, 47-month study of safety and efficacy of calcium hydroxylapatite for soft tissue augmentation of nasolabial folds and other areas of the face. Dermatol Surg 2007; 33(Suppl 2):S122–6 [discussion: S126–7].

18. Onesti MG, Troccola A, Scuderi N. Volumetric correction using poly-L-lactic acid in facial asymmetry: Parry Romberg syndrome and scleroderma. Dermatol Surg 2009;35(9):1368–75.

19. Palm MD, Woodhall KE, Butterwick KJ, et al. Cosmetic use of poly-l-lactic acid: a retrospective study of 130 patients. Dermatol Surg 2010;36(2): 161–70.

20. Cohen S, Dover J, Monheit G, et al. Five-year safety and satisfaction study of PMMA-Collagen in the correction of nasolabial folds. Dermatol Surg 2015; 41(Suppl 1):S302–13.

Noninvasive Body Contouring
A Male Perspective

Heidi Wat, MD[a], Douglas C. Wu, MD, PhD[b],*,
Mitchel P. Goldman, MD[b]

KEYWORDS

- Body contouring • V-taper • Jawline • Cryolipolysis

KEY POINTS

- Noninvasive body contouring is an attractive therapeutic modality to enhance the ideal male physique.
- An understanding of the body contour men strive for allows the treating physician to focus on areas that are of most concern to men.
- Patients of physicians with an understanding of body counter have an enhanced experience.

INTRODUCTION

The male cosmetic patient tends to gravitate toward treatments that require minimal downtime, involve minimal discomfort, and be associated with no visually apparent side effects. In the realm of body contouring, men place higher value on enhancing a well-defined, strong, masculine jawline and developing a V-shaped taper through the upper body. To achieve this contour, the areas of focus are the submental region, the male chest, the abdomen, and the flanks (**Fig. 1**). Contouring of the lower body, including thighs, knees, and calves, is of lesser importance to men who tend not to develop excessive adiposity in those areas and are typically more interested in developing muscle mass. In this review, we discuss noninvasive body contouring techniques while taking into account the unique aesthetic concerns of the male patient by combining an analysis of the existing literature with our own clinical experience.

SUBMENTAL AND JAWLINE CONTOURING
Cryolipolysis

Cryolipolysis relies on adipocyte response to acute cold injury by inducing a lobular panniculitis, which results in subcutaneous fat layer reduction. Initial proof of concept studies were performed in porcine models with tissue temperatures typically below the freezing point.[1,2] Subsequent clinical work revealed that treatment efficacy is achieved at skin surface temperatures between 10°C and 17°C and subcutaneous fat temperatures between 9°C and 14°C.[3] Cryolipolysis is now widely performed on a large variety of anatomic sites.[4] The male aesthetic patient, however, typically tends to focus on the submentum, the abdomen, the flanks, and the breast. Indeed, clinical trials involving cryolipolysis to otherwise common areas, such as the medial and lateral thighs and the posterior upper arms, have typically lacked male participation even though this population was not directly excluded.[5–7]

Disclosure: The authors have nothing they wish to disclose.
[a] Division of Dermatology, Department of Medicine, University of Alberta, 13-103 Clinical Sciences Building, 11350-83 Avenue, Edmonton, Alberta T6G 2G3, Canada; [b] Goldman, Butterwick, Groff, Fabi, and Wu Cosmetic Laser Dermatology, San Diego, CA, USA
* Corresponding author. 9339 Genesee Avenue, Suite 300, San Diego, CA 92121.
E-mail address: dwu@clderm.com

derm.theclinics.com

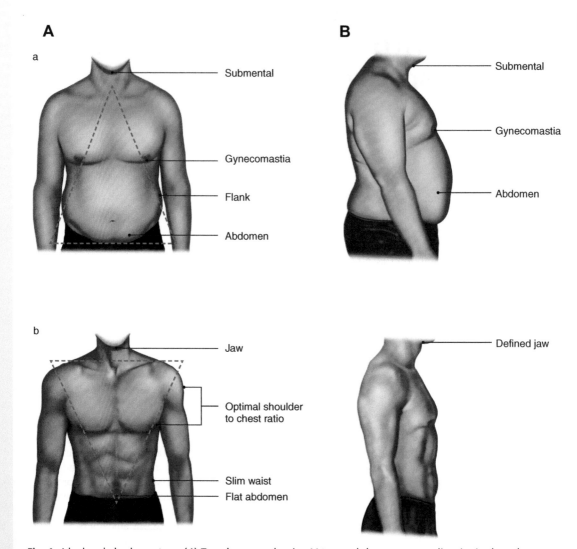

Fig. 1. Ideal male body contour. (*A*) To enhance a pleasing V-tapered shape, excess adiposity in the submentum, chest, abdomen, and flanks (*a*) should be reduced (*b*). (*B*) Side profile.

Excess adiposity in the submental region is a common concern among men. An aesthetically pleasing masculine jawline strongly demarcates the lower face from the neck, and excess submental fat is obscuring. Two prospective clinical trials examining the safety and efficacy of cryolipolysis in this region have been performed with a cumulative male subject proportion of 19% (14 of 74).[8,9] In both trials, one to two treatment cycles were performed 6 weeks apart with a 3-month follow-up. Subjects were generally pleased. Ultrasound measurements detected a roughly 2-mm fat layer reduction.

Synthetic Sodium Deoxycholic Acid

Another option for male submental contouring is injectable synthetic sodium deoxycholate (SDOC). SDOC disrupts adipocyte cell membranes leading to cell death and a subsequent inflammatory response that clears cellular debris. Four phase III randomized, double-blind, placebo-controlled clinical trials have examined the safety and efficacy of SDOC for the reduction of unwanted submental fat.[10–13] These trials included a total of 1744 subjects of which 194 were men who received SDOC (11.1%). Subjects were treated up to 6 times with treatment intervals of 28 days. The results uniformly demonstrated significant submental fat reduction and increased patient satisfaction in the active treatment arm versus placebo. The percentage of subjects who achieved a one-point or greater reduction in submental fat score ranged from 50% to 70% with SDOC versus 20% to 30% with placebo. Two of these trials performed MRI assessment of submental fat reduction[12,13] and found that 40% to 46% of SDOC-treated subjects achieved a 10% volumetric reduction versus 5% with placebo. No increased skin laxity was detected posttreatment.

Successful application of injectable SDOC for submental contouring is heavily dependent on appropriate patient selection. Good candidates for treatment exhibit submental fullness caused by excess subcutaneous fat rather than other causes, such as thyromegaly or lymphadenopathy; do not exhibit excessive platysmal banding or skin laxity; and have not had previous surgical treatments in the area that may complicate subsequent SDOC therapy.[14] Management of patient expectations is also critical because multiple treatment sessions over an extended period of time are typically required to achieve optimal outcomes. Furthermore, unavoidable side effects, such as pain, bruising, and significant edema during and posttreatment, must be fully explained. Simple measures, such as oral ibuprofen or coinjection of lidocaine, can reduce treatment pain.[15,16] Additionally, in our experience, mixing a small amount of triamcinaolone with the SDOC (1–2 mg/mL) produces a significant decrease in pain and treatment-related edema without compromising treatment efficacy.

Subsurface Monopolar Radiofrequency

Subsurface monopolar radiofrequency is a minimally invasive technique that is designed to simultaneous reduce excessive submental adiposity and tighten loose skin of the neck and jawline. The proper application of this technology has the potential to enhance a strong and defined male jawline. By applying heat at temperatures of 55°C to 70°C to the dermal-epidermal junction and subcutaneous fat while maintaining an epidermal surface temperature below 46°C, adipocyte necrosis, dermal neocollagenesis, and epidermal sparing are achieved. Prospective clinical trials involving men using subsurface monopolar radiofrequency have not been published. Two retrospective studies with 17% male participation reported good clinical efficacy and safety.[17,18] In our experience, subsurface monopolar radiofrequency for contouring of the neck and jawline is a pleasing minimally invasive therapeutic option in men.

ENHANCEMENT OF THE V-TAPER

A pleasing V-tapered male body contour relies on an ideal shoulder to chest ratio; a slim waist; and a flat, defined abdomen. This ideal is enhanced by reducing male pseudogynecomastia and unwanted flank and central abdominal fat.

Pseudogynecomastia

One anatomic site that is exclusively a concern among men is the excessive male breast. Pseudogynecomastia is the benign enlargement of the male breast caused by excess subareolar fat. This unwanted fullness tends to be accentuated in the inferior aspect of the male chest, obscuring the ideal V-taper by decreasing the shoulder to chest ratio. Munavalli and Panchaprateep[19] treated 21 men for pseudogynecomastia. Following two treatments, 95% of subjects reported improved visual appearance and 89% reported reduced embarrassment associated with their condition. Additionally, ultrasound measurements detected a mean fat layer reduction of 1.6 mm ± 1.2 mm. We performed a split-breast study in 10 male subjects with pseudogynecomastia and found an 8.12 mm ± 6.94 mm versus a 1.03 mm ± 6.03 mm fat layer reduction by ultrasound measurement in the treated versus untreated breast at 6 weeks post–single cryolipolysis treatment ($P = .03$; Jones and colleagues, unpublished data). Mean patient satisfaction was significantly higher for the treated breast versus the untreated breast (**Fig. 2**). Treatment in this area tends to be well tolerated, although one of the subjects in our trial withdrew because of pain and one subject in the Munavalli trial experienced paradoxic adipose hyperplasia (PAH).

Reduction of Abdominal and Flank Girth

Reducing frontal abdominal protrusion and narrowing of the waist are of paramount importance to men seeking noninvasive body contouring. These areas remain the focus of most noninvasive body contouring technologies including cryolipolysis, nonthermal focused ultrasound, high-intensity thermal focused ultrasound (HIFU), and focus field radiofrequency.

Cryolipolysis

The safety and efficacy of cryolipolysis to the abdomen and flanks is well-documented. There

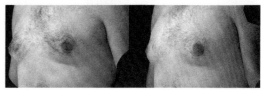

Fig. 2. Before and after cryolipolysis to the male breast.

are seven prospective clinical trials that have included male subjects.[3,20–25] The cumulative proportion of male subjects was 30% (38 of 127). Fat layer thickness was reduced by 14% to 20% via caliper measurement after one to two treatment sessions corresponding to roughly 40 mL of volumetric loss.[20,21,24] In our experience, cryolipolysis to the abdomen and flanks in the male population is an effective and pleasing treatment (**Fig. 3**). When evaluating male patients for this procedure, particular attention should be paid to the degree of subcutaneous versus visceral fat that is present because cryolipolysis has shown no efficacy in the reduction of visceral abdominal fat.[24]

Adverse events secondary to cryolipolysis tend to be mild and transient, potentially consisting of erythema, edema, bruising, tenderness, and skin numbness.[26,27] Two rarer side effects have been reported in the literature: delayed pain and PAH. Keaney and colleagues[28] performed a retrospective analysis of 125 patients who received 554 cryolipolysis treatments to analyze variables that may influence the development of delayed posttreatment pain. In this study, risk factors identified included young age (mean, 39 years), female gender, and abdominal treatment area. However, all cases of delayed pain were self-limited and resolved within 3 to 11 days without long-term sequelae. Management of this phenomenon includes mild analgesics, such as lidocaine 5% transdermal patch; gabapentin, 300 mg twice daily; and/or acetaminophen with codeine.

PAH is an even rarer potential adverse side effect of cryolipolysis with an estimated incidence of 1 in 20,000.[29] It is thought to be more common in men with potential risk factors including excessive visceral abdominal fat and the presence of firm, nondistensible, fibrous fat within the treatment area.[30] However, further studies are required to isolate the true cause and consequence of PAH following cryolipolysis. Tumescent liposculpture has been suggested as a possible treatment modality for PAH, although a recent case was reported refractory to even this technique.[31]

Radiofrequency

Contactless focused field radiofrequency has demonstrated safety and efficacy in the treatment of excess abdominal girth in men (**Fig. 4**). This technology operates on the principle of oscillating electromagnetic fields that force collisions between charged ions causing the production of heat. When applied specifically to the subcutaneous fat layer, adipose tissue temperatures reach 45°C while skin temperatures remain below 40°C. This selective heating leads to adipocyte apoptosis while sparing the overlying skin.[32] Three prospective clinical trials have been performed assessing the ability of focused field radiofrequency to reduce abdominal circumference.[33–35] A cumulative total of 60 subjects were treated, of which 13 were men (22%). After a series of weekly treatment sessions, these trials demonstrated a 3-cm abdominal circumferential reduction,[33] 5.36-mm reduction in subcutaneous fat layer thickness by MRI,[34] and a 4.17-mm reduction by ultrasound examination[35] at 1 to 3 months post final treatment session. Although the study populations were small, the preclinical and clinical data to date suggest that focused field radiofrequency is a viable therapeutic option for the reduction of unwanted abdominal girth in men. Of note, two clinical trials with this technology have been performed for the contouring of the thigh but of the 82 subjects enrolled, none were men suggesting that this is not an area of high cosmetic concern for men who have an interest in noninvasive body contouring.[36,37]

Ultrasound

The use of ultrasound technology for noninvasive body contouring is divided into nonthermal,

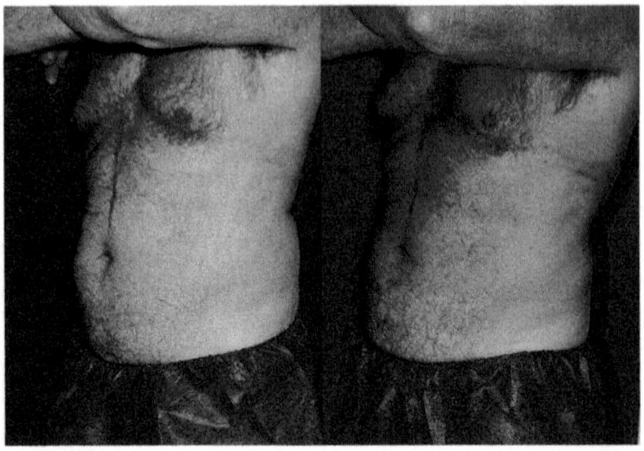

Fig. 3. Before and after cryolipolysis to the abdomen and flanks.

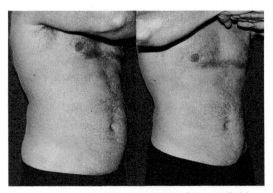

Fig. 4. Before and after contactless focused field radiofrequency of abdomen and flanks.

low-frequency focused ultrasound, and HIFU. Nonthermal focused ultrasound relies on the oscillation and disruption of adipocyte membranes leading to cell death, whereas HIFU transforms ultrasound energy into heat thus leading to adipocyte necrosis. Low-frequency ultrasound delivers mainly mechanical energy that results in cavitation when the negative acoustic pressure supersedes adipocyte membrane adhesion.[38] High-frequency, high-intensity ultrasound produces instantaneous heating of tissues to 55°C to 70°C and results in coagulative necrosis of adipocytes while sparing surrounding tissues and preserving epidermal integrity.[39] In terms of noninvasive body contouring, both technologies have been primarily studied for the reduction of unwanted subcutaneous abdominal fat, although HIFU has also been applied to the ablation of uterine fibroids and nephrolithiasis.

There are four prospective clinical trials studying nonthermal focused ultrasound for abdominal contouring that included men.[40–43] A total of 397 subjects were studied with 76 being men (19%). Three of the four clinical trials demonstrated safety and efficacy of this technology[40–42] with circumferential reductions measured between 1 cm and 4 cm. However, the lone Asian trial failed to demonstrate efficacy of nonthermal focused ultrasound in this patient population.[43] Further work may be required in select patient populations, but overall this technology seems to be safe and effective in reducing unwanted subcutaneous abdominal fat. Because of its nonthermal nature, treatments also tend to be painless and with minimal to no side effects. This is especially attractive to the male cosmetic patient who tends to gravitate toward treatments that require minimal downtime, involve minimal discomfort, and be associated with no visually apparent side effects.

HIFU was first studied for noninvasive ablation of subcutaneous fat in 2009.[44] Six studies looking at the use of HIFU for treatment of abdomen and flanks included male participants. The cumulative proportion of male patients was 18.2 (108 of 592).[45–50] Studies consistently demonstrated mean reduction in waist circumference of 2.06 cm to 2.51 cm after a single treatment at 12-week follow-up. Cumulative energies used ranged from 104 J/cm² to 180 J/cm² delivered over two to three passes One of the earlier retrospecttive case series published by Fatemi and Kane[45] demonstrated a much higher mean waist circumference reduction of 4.6 cm ± 2.4 cm after a single treatment. In this study, the mean cumulative energy used was 134.8 J/cm² delivered over two passes. The only randomized sham controlled trial compared high-energy (59 J/cm² × 3 passes = 177 J/cm²) and low-energy (47 J/cm² × 3 passes = 141 J/cm²) treatment with sham treatment. At 12-week follow-up, only the high-energy group demonstrated a statistically significant waist circumference reduction of 2.06 cm and higher patient satisfaction compared with sham treatment in the intention-to-treat analysis. However, there was an 8.9% dropout rate, which is fairly high for these types of studies. If these patients were excluded in a per protocol analysis, high- and low-energy treatment groups were significantly improved from sham treatment. Subsequent studies by Robinson and colleagues[49] and Shek and colleagues[20] showed that overall efficacy seems to be determined by cumulative fluence rather than fluence per pass or stacking technique. Robinson and colleagues[49] conducted a multicenter trial comparing 30 J/cm² to 60 J/cm² per pass, 150 J/cm² versus 180 J/cm² cumulative fluence, and a grid repeat versus site repeat treatment pattern and showed no significant difference between the treatment groups. There was a mean 2.3 cm ± 2.9 cm waist circumference reduction at 12 weeks. However, pain was significantly higher in the 60 J/cm² protocols. Shek and colleagues similarly demonstrated a 2.1-cm waist circumference reduction using lower fluences per pass (30–55 J/cm²) on Asian patients. Fluence per pass was adjusted based on pain levels, and 55 J/cm² seemed to be the ceiling for most patients.[20] Typically lower fluences are used if a greater number of passes are delivered to achieve equivalent efficacy.

Adverse effects include pain, ecchymosis, edema, erythema, and dysesthesia that are self-limited. Pain is often tolerable with standard oral analgesics. A safety and tolerability split-abdomen study showed mean pain scores (0–10) of 3.5 ± 2.3 in treated side compared with 0.17 ± 0.41 on sham treated side.[51] Cholesterol, triglycerides, liver enzymes, complete blood count, and inflammatory markers remained unchanged at Day 1, 3, 7, and 14 posttreatment.[51]

HIFU is an excellent treatment option for males seeking reduction in waist circumference with minimal pain and adverse sequelae. Mean reductions in waist circumference are similar to cyrolipolysis. A small study comparing HIFU with cryolipolysis by our group also found comparable efficacy with substantially more pain and bruising with HIFU.[52]

SUMMARY

Noninvasive body contouring is an attractive therapeutic modality to enhance the ideal male physique. An understanding of the body contour men strive for allows the treating physician to focus on areas that are of most concern to men, thus enhancing patient experience and satisfaction.

REFERENCES

1. Manstein D, Laubach H, Watanabe K, et al. Selective cryolysis: a novel method of non-invasive fat removal. Lasers Surg Med 2008;40(9):595–604.
2. Zelickson B, Egbert BM, Preciado J, et al. Cryolipolysis for noninvasive fat cell destruction: initial results from a pig model. Dermatol Surg 2009;35(10):1462–70.
3. Sasaki GH, Abelev N, Tevez-Ortiz A. Noninvasive selective cryolipolysis and reperfusion recovery for localized natural fat reduction and contouring. Aesthet Surg J 2014;34(3):420–31.
4. Avram MM, Harry RS. Cryolipolysis for subcutaneous fat layer reduction. Lasers Surg Med 2009;41(10):703–8.
5. Stevens WG, Bachelor EP. Cryolipolysis conformable-surface applicator for nonsurgical fat reduction in lateral thighs. Aesthet Surg J 2015;35(1):66–71.
6. Zelickson BD, Burns AJ, Kilmer SL. Cryolipolysis for safe and effective inner thigh fat reduction. Lasers Surg Med 2015;47(2):120–7.
7. Lee SJ, Jang HW, Kim H, et al. Non-invasive cryolipolysis to reduce subcutaneous fat in the arms. J Cosmet Laser Ther 2016;18(3):126–9.
8. Kilmer SL, Burns AJ, Zelickson BD. Safety and efficacy of cryolipolysis for non-invasive reduction of submental fat. Lasers Surg Med 2016;48(1):3–13.
9. Bernstein EF, Bloom JD. Safety and efficacy of bilateral submental cryolipolysis with quantified 3-dimensional imaging of fat reduction and skin tightening. JAMA Facial Plast Surg 2017;19(5):350–7.
10. Ascher B, Hoffmann K, Walker P, et al. Efficacy, patient-reported outcomes and safety profile of ATX-101 (deoxycholic acid), an injectable drug for the reduction of unwanted submental fat: results from a phase III, randomized, placebo-controlled study. J Eur Acad Dermatol Venereol 2014;28(12):1707–15.
11. Rzany B, Griffiths T, Walker P, et al. Reduction of unwanted submental fat with ATX-101 (deoxycholic acid), an adipocytolytic injectable treatment: results from a phase III, randomized, placebo-controlled study. Br J Dermatol 2014;170(2):445–53.
12. Humphrey S, Sykes J, Kantor J, et al. ATX-101 for reduction of submental fat: a phase III randomized controlled trial. J Am Acad Dermatol Oct 2016;75(4):788–97.e7.
13. Jones DH, Carruthers J, Joseph JH, et al. REFINE-1, a multicenter, randomized, double-blind, placebo-controlled, phase 3 trial with ATX-101, an injectable drug for submental fat reduction. Dermatol Surg 2016;42(1):38–49.
14. Jones DH, Kenkel JM, Fagien S, et al. Proper technique for administration of ATX-101 (deoxycholic acid injection): insights from an injection practicum and roundtable discussion. Dermatol Surg 2016;42(Suppl 1):S275–81.
15. Dover JS, Kenkel JM, Carruthers A, et al. Management of patient experience with ATX-101 (deoxycholic acid injection) for reduction of submental fat. Dermatol Surg 2016;42(Suppl 1):S288–99.
16. Humphrey S. Management of patient experience with ATX-101 (deoxycholic acid injection) for reduction of submental fat. Dermatol Surg 2016;42(12):1397–8.
17. Dendle J, Wu DC, Fabi SG, et al. A retrospective evaluation of subsurface monopolar radiofrequency for lifting of the face, neck, and jawline. Dermatol Surg 2016;42(11):1261–5.
18. Key DJ. Integration of thermal imaging with subsurface radiofrequency thermistor heating for the purpose of skin tightening and contour improvement: a retrospective review of clinical efficacy. J Drugs Dermatol 2014;13(12):1485–9.
19. Munavalli GS, Panchaprateep R. Cryolipolysis for targeted fat reduction and improved appearance of the enlarged male breast. Dermatol Surg 2015;41(9):1043–51.
20. Shek SY, Chan NP, Chan HH. Non-invasive cryolipolysis for body contouring in Chinese: a first commercial experience. Lasers Surg Med 2012;44(2):125–30.
21. Garibyan L, Sipprell WH 3rd, Jalian HR, et al. Three-dimensional volumetric quantification of fat loss following cryolipolysis. Lasers Surg Med 2014;46(2):75–80.
22. Kim J, Kim DH, Ryu HJ. Clinical effectiveness of non-invasive selective cryolipolysis. J Cosmet Laser Ther 2014;16(5):209–13.
23. Few J, Gold M, Sadick N. Prospective internally controlled blind reviewed clinical evaluation of cryolipolysis combined with multipolar radiofrequency andvaripulsetechnology for enhanced subject results in circumferential fat reduction and skin laxity of the flanks. J Drugs Dermatol 2016;15(11):1354–8.
24. Mostafa MS, Elshafey MA. Cryolipolysis versus laser lipolysis on adolescent abdominal adiposity. Lasers Surg Med 2016;48(4):365–70.
25. Kilmer SL. Prototype CoolCup cryolipolysis applicator with over 40% reduced treatment time demonstrates equivalent safety and efficacy with greater patient preference. Lasers Surg Med 2017;49(1):63–8.
26. Vanaman M, Fabi SG, Carruthers J. Complications in the cosmetic dermatology patient: a review and our experience (part 1). Dermatol Surg 2016;42(1):1–11.

27. Vanaman M, Fabi SG, Carruthers J. Complications in the cosmetic dermatology patient: a review and our experience (part 2). Dermatol Surg 2016;42(1):12–20.

28. Keaney TC, Gudas AT, Alster TS. Delayed Onset pain associated with cryolipolysis treatment: a retrospective study with treatment recommendations. Dermatol Surg 2015;41(11):1296–9.

29. Jalian HR, Avram MM, Garibyan L, et al. Paradoxical adipose hyperplasia after cryolipolysis. JAMA Dermatol 2014;150(3):317–9.

30. Keaney TC, Naga LI. Men at risk for paradoxical adipose hyperplasia after cryolipolysis. J Cosmet Dermatol 2016;15(4):575–7.

31. Friedmann DP, Buckley S, Mishra V. Paradoxical adipose hyperplasia after cryoadipolysis refractory to tumescent liposuction. Dermatol Surg 2017;43(8):1103–5.

32. McDaniel D, Lozanova P. Human adipocyte apoptosis immediately following high frequency focused field radio frequency: case study. J Drugs Dermatol 2015;14(6):622–3.

33. Pumprla J, Howorka K, Kolackova Z, et al. Noncontact radiofrequency-induced reduction of subcutaneous abdominal fat correlates with initial cardiovascular autonomic balance and fat tissue hormones: safety analysis. F1000Res 2015;4:49.

34. Downie J, Kaspar M. Contactless abdominal fat reduction with selective RF evaluated by magnetic resonance imaging (MRI): case study. J Drugs Dermatol 2016;15(4):491–5.

35. Hayre N, Palm M, Jenkin P. A clinical evaluation of a next generation, non-invasive, selective radiofrequency, hands-free, body-shaping device. J Drugs Dermatol 2016;15(12):1557–61.

36. McDaniel D, Samkova P. Evaluation of the safety and efficacy of a non-contact radiofrequency device for the improvement in contour and circumferential reduction of the inner and outer thigh. J Drugs Dermatol 2015;14(12):1422–4.

37. Fritz K, Samkova P, Salavastru C, et al. A novel selective RF applicator for reducing thigh circumference: a clinical evaluation. Dermatol Ther 2016;29(2):92–5.

38. Jewell ML, Solish NJ, Desilets CS. Noninvasive body sculpting technologies with an emphasis on high-intensity focused ultrasound. Aesthetic Plast Surg 2011;35(5):901–12.

39. Jewell ML, Desilets C, Smoller BR. Evaluation of a novel high-intensity focused ultrasound device: pre-clinical studies in a porcine model. Aesthet Surg J 2011;31(4):429–34.

40. Moreno-Moraga J, Valero-Altes T, Riquelme AM, et al. Body contouring by non-invasive transdermal focused ultrasound. Lasers Surg Med 2007;39(4):315–23.

41. Teitelbaum SA, Burns JL, Kubota J, et al. Noninvasive body contouring by focused ultrasound: safety and efficacy of the Contour I device in a multicenter, controlled, clinical study. Plast Reconstr Surg 2007;120(3):779–89 [discussion: 790].

42. Coleman WP 3rd, Coleman W 4th, Weiss RA, et al. A multicenter controlled study to evaluate multiple treatments with nonthermal focused ultrasound for noninvasive fat reduction. Dermatol Surg 2017;43(1):50–7.

43. Shek S, Yu C, Yeung CK, et al. The use of focused ultrasound for non-invasive body contouring in Asians. Lasers Surg Med 2009;41(10):751–9.

44. Fatemi A. High-intensity focused ultrasound effectively reduces adipose tissue. Semin Cutan Med Surg 2009;28(4):257–62.

45. Fatemi A, Kane MA. High-intensity focused ultrasound effectively reduces waist circumference by ablating adipose tissue from the abdomen and flanks: a retrospective case series. Aesthetic Plast Surg 2010;34(5):577–82.

46. Gadsden E, Aguilar MT, Smoller BR, et al. Evaluation of a novel high-intensity focused ultrasound device for ablating subcutaneous adipose tissue for noninvasive body contouring: safety studies in human volunteers. Aesthet Surg J 2011;31(4):401–10.

47. Jewell ML, Baxter RA, Cox SE, et al. Randomized sham-controlled trial to evaluate the safety and effectiveness of a high-intensity focused ultrasound device for noninvasive body sculpting. Plast Reconstr Surg 2011;128(1):253–62.

48. Solish N, Lin X, Axford-Gatley RA, et al. A randomized, single-blind, postmarketing study of multiple energy levels of high-intensity focused ultrasound for noninvasive body sculpting. Dermatol Surg 2012;38(1):58–67.

49. Robinson DM, Kaminer MS, Baumann L, et al. High-intensity focused ultrasound for the reduction of subcutaneous adipose tissue using multiple treatment techniques. Dermatol Surg 2014;40(6):641–51.

50. Shek SY, Yeung CK, Chan JC, et al. Efficacy of high-intensity focused ultrasonography for noninvasive body sculpting in Chinese patients. Lasers Surg Med 2014;46(4):263–9.

51. Shalom A, Wiser I, Brawer S, et al. Safety and tolerability of a focused ultrasound device for treatment of adipose tissue in subjects undergoing abdominoplasty: a placebo-control pilot study. Dermatol Surg 2013;39(5):744–51.

52. Friedmann D, Mahoney L, Fabi S, et al. A pilot prospective comparative trial of high-intensity focused ultrasound versus cryolipolysis for flank subcutaneous adipose tissue and review of the literature. Cosmet Dermatol 2013;30:152–8.

Advances in Hair Restoration

Paul T. Rose, MD, JD

KEYWORDS

- Robotic surgery • FUE • PRP • Scalp micropigmentation • Stem cells • Low-level light lasers
- Hair graft survival

KEY POINTS

- Selection of hair transplantation methodology depends on patient's goals, type of hair loss, and quality of hair.
- Robotic hair transplantation is the latest frontier in hair restoration.
- Platelet-rich plasma, low-level laser therapy, and stem cells can be used together with hair transplantation to enhance graft survival.

INTRODUCTION

Modern hair transplantation is based on the use of naturally occurring hair groupings referred to as follicular units (FUs)[1] These FUs may be acquired with the use of strip harvesting or the extraction of the FUs with a small punch, generally 0.8 mm to 1.2 mm in diameter.

The decision as to how the grafts should be obtained will vary with each individual patient and their particular needs at the time of surgery. Each technique has advantages and disadvantages. The process of hair restoration continues to be refined in an effort to create better cosmetic results, growth of hair, and preservation of existing hair. The advances that we are witnessing in hair restoration are occurring in several areas. These include technological advances in recovering grafts and placing grafts, bio-enhancements with storage media and intraoperative manipulation, and adjunctive treatments.

In this article we discuss many of the latest advances in hair restoration.

Technological Advances

For the past several years, a robotic modality for harvesting grafts has been available.[2,3] This device (Artas; Restoration Robotics, Sunnyvale, CA) harvest grafts using a double-needle apparatus that is controlled through the use of a video camera system. Since the initial iteration, this device has been shown to harvest FU extraction (FUE) grafts very reliably. The newest software update is reported to permit harvesting at rates of more than 1500 grafts per hour with low transection rates. The system allows for the use of smaller needles, ranging in size from 0.8 mm to 1 mm and different needle designs to suit various situations. It may be that smaller needles could create smaller wounds in terms of eventual healing.

An improved lighting system enables the operating staff to more easily visualize the operative field and access the grafts for removal within the grids as the machine is functioning. The latest software allows the robot to assess the area to be harvested within a grid and with a single-button, one-touch system the device can ascertain the potential graft positions within the grid rather than having the operator manipulate the device to position it properly. The robotic head has undergone a design change that facilitates greater ease of movement of the device without having to shift the patient.

Disclosure Statement: P.T. Rose is a consultant and shareholder in Restoration Robotics.
Hair Transplant Institute of Miami, Offices of Merrick Park, 4425 Ponce de Leon Boulevard, Suite 230, Coral Gables, FL 33146, USA
E-mail address: paultrose@yahoo.com

Dermatol Clin 36 (2018) 57–62
https://doi.org/10.1016/j.det.2017.09.008

The algorithm for harvesting allows the operator to differentiate 1-hair, 2-hair, and 3-hair grafts and the ability to select these to harvest. In terms of making recipient sites, the new software permits the creation of recipient angles of 35° and is most helpful in making sites on the top/horizontal aspect of the scalp. It should be noted that this program may not be optimal in making sites at the lateral aspects of the scalp.

The robotic system has an integrated design feature that can allow the surgeon to draw out a hairline and the area to be transplanted. This design pattern can be transferred to the patient and followed by the robot in making recipient sites. Many physicians prefer to make the hairline sites themselves before considering using the site making mode. The author still prefers to make his own sites throughout the recipient area.

As with any approach to surgery, the robotic device is not perfect for all patients, and the surgeon must select patients who will benefit most from this approach. The author has found that patients with fine hair, thin skin, and very mobile skin can be less well suited for treatment with the robotic device.

Several new drills have been developed to which FUE punches can be attached. One drill in particular has been well received. The WAW (Devroye Instruments, Brussels, Belgium) uses an oscillating mechanism to facilitate the extraction of grafts. A foot pedal with 3 dials controls the initial speed of rotation, degree of oscillation, and speed of oscillation.[4]

In addition, Dr Devroye has developed a punch that he refers to as a "trumpet punch."[4] This punch is constructed so that the inner bore of the punch is sloped and blunted to facilitate obtaining grafts and the external border is flat and sharp. The blunt internal border aids in avoiding transection.

It is advised that the surgeon use light pressure to allow the sharp edge to enter the epidermis initially and then allow for the oscillation to begin before venturing deeper into the tissue.

Other developments with punches include the hex punch from Dr Harris.[5] The hex design acts to disrupt the tissue around the graft using vibratory action, which allows easier removal of the FU with less transection as compared with other punches.

A slotted punch developed by the author[6] originally to facilitate visualization of hair angles and proper centering for FUE harvesting, has been adapted by Drs Park and Boaventura[7,8] to allow for harvesting of long hair grafts.

The process of long hair harvesting allows the patient to avoid shaving large areas of donor. The slotted punch technique for long hair is quite tedious and there can be higher rates of transection.

Usually small areas in various parts of the donor area are shaved and the grafts are taken from these areas. This allows the patient to cover any evidence of the surgical process.

Implantation

Traditionally the primary approach to placing grafts has been the use of jeweler's forceps to grasp the FU grafts and then place them into the recipient sites. To do this proficiently can involve substantial practice. Holding the grafts too tightly can lead to damage to the grafts and repeated attempts to place the grafts can also lead to damage. This may be a factor in some poor growth outcomes.

Increasingly, clinicians are adopting the use of implanters to aid in placing grafts. There are multiple implanters on the market, such as the Lion (Hans Biomed, Korea), OKT (Choi Instruments, Korea), and others, but the basic design is similar.[9–11] A needlelike cylinder with a slit is attached to a spring-loaded stem that can push a graft into the skin after the implanter has been appropriately loaded. Sharp implanters are used to make the recipient site and place the grafts at the same time. Some surgeons are blunting the tips of the implanters and use the implanters after sites have been created.[12] It is felt that the use of this type of implanter allows for less trauma during graft insertion. The technique uses premade sites that can be sagittal or coronal. Currently the surgeon must make or have someone else take a sharp implanter and make the tip dull. This is accomplished by using sandpaper such as 400 or 600 g weight paper and rubbing it over the edge of the needle of the implanter until it is sufficiently blunted.

Implanters come in various needle sizes to accommodate differing graft sizes. The surgeon must select the appropriate size to be used, and if there is difficulty placing the graft, repeated manipulation may damage the grafts. Many implanters are re-useable and can be taken apart, cleaned, and then sterilized for reuse.

An important aspect of the use of implanters is the work flow that must occur to perform implantation efficiently.[11] In general, there must be at least 1 person loading the grafts, a second person handing the grafts to the surgeon to implant, and that person must then receive the unloaded implanter and pass it back to the loader. This system can take considerable time to develop. If the surgeon attempts to use 2 people implanting, this adds more complexity.

Bio-Enhancements

In an effort to improve graft survival, hair transplant surgeons are increasingly using bio-enhancements to decrease reperfusion injury and maintain energy for the cells of the grafts. The surgeon should be aware that the hair transplant grafts are without a blood supply for several days. The cells acquire nutrients via the process of inosculation. It can take 3 to 5 days for the graft to obtain a blood supply.

Some physicians are using more physiologic storage media such as Hypothermosol (Biolife, Seattle, WA).[13,14] As grafts have no blood supply and are often stored out of the body for several hours, the tissue is subject to the effects of thermal damage, ischemia, reperfusion injury, and a lack of necessary nutrients, such as ATP, glucose, and oxygen. The normal balance between extracellular milieu and intracellular milieu can be adversely altered as the membrane ion pumps can be disrupted. Osmotic and oncotic imbalance can ensue, which is detrimental to cellular survival. Additionally, free radicals that would normally be eliminated with antioxidants may build up.

In an effort to respond to the metabolic needs of these grafts, a medium such as Hypothermosol can act to maintain ionic and osmotic balance, aid and support cellular metabolism, assist in the removal of free radicals, and ultimately decrease cellular death. This material storage medium has been shown to reduce apoptosis and diminish reperfusion injury.[14] Hypothermosol is designed to be used at lower temperatures of 2 to 8°C, and in hair graft storage, lower temperature storage is used to decrease cellular energy requirements.

Studies on the use of hyperthermosol are limited, but they suggest an increase in graft survival and there are anecdotal reports of better graft growth and earlier growth.

Recently the use of liposomal-encased ATP as an addition to the storage medium and as an adjunct in postoperative healing sprays has been advocated.[14]

A liposomal-encased ATP (Energy Delivery Solutions, Jeffersonville, IN) has been developed and this is the primary product in use. Again, studies are limited but there is a perception that this helps in graft survival. Studies in animals have shown that the addition of ATP can preserve limbs that have been amputated and reattached. As hair grafts are without supplemental oxygen while in holding solutions, the injury from ischemia could harm grafts and ultimately graft survival by protecting the ischemic cells. The use of ATP compensates for this period of lack of oxygenation by providing energy to the cells. The ATP also acts as a vasodilator, bringing in additional nutrients and decreasing reperfusion injury. The use of liposomal ATP also has been suggested as a postoperative spray, as it takes 4 to 5 days for a hair graft to be rebuild a vascular supply.

We use the combination of Hypothermosol and ATP in our practice as a holding solution. A common recipe for the use of Hypothermosol and ATP is 1 mL ATP to 100 mL Hypothermosol.

Adjuncts to Hair Transplant Surgery

Platelet-rich plasma

The use of platelet-rich plasma (PRP) for many maladies is rapidly growing. It is commonly used in orthopedic injuries, wound healing, dental procedures, and cosmetic facial procedures.[15,16] The use of PRP for the medical treatment of hair loss is also increasing but it is also being used during the surgical process.[17] The author uses it for the donor area of strip harvest cases, as well as the wounds created by FUE, and routinely we use it in the recipient area.

The alpha granules of platelets are known to release various growth factors. These include vascular endothelial growth factor, insulinlike growth factor, epidermal growth factor, fibroblast growth factor, and others. In vitro studies on mice with the use of human PRP have shown positive responses and stimulation of hair growth.[18–23]

Studies in humans are generally positive, but a recent study in a woman with androgenetic alopecia did not show a positive response.[24] This leads to an important aspect of evaluating the efficacy of PRP. There are many different PRP systems available. Some use a single spin with the centrifuge, whereas other preparations require 2 spins. Spin times and spin force can also vary. There are PRP systems that use activation of PRP with calcium chloride or calcium gluconate, whereas other systems use nonactivated PRP.

We are at a point where clinicians need to be able to more rationally compare various PRP products and the studies related to PRP usage.

Many systems are available for producing PRP and the literature is generally encouraging as to the positive effects of PRP. The use of PRP for wound healing is well established, so it seems very reasonable to use PRP for the donor strip wounds as well as for FUE wounds to enhance healing. Many surgeons when using PRP during hair transplantation will use some of the material for the recipient area and some will "dip" or bathe the grafts in PRP before implantation. There is anecdotal evidence that the use of PRP in these instances can increase graft survival and possibly allow closer packing of grafts.

What is concerning about the use of PRP is a lack of protocols and an adequate understanding of what the parameters for injection of this material should be.

The author is currently using a 2-spin system at 3500 rpm that reliably provides 3 to 6 times the baseline concentration of platelets. We measure the baseline and the PRP concentration to see if we have adequately concentrated the PRP.

We are using PRP as a preprocedure adjunct as well as during a hair transplant procedure. In our facility, the use of PRP has proved beneficial for improving atrophic scalp tissue, donor wound healing, alopecia areata, diffuse alopecia, and telogen effluvium.

At times we have added a porcine matrix (Acell, Matristem, NJ) to serve as a "scaffold" for the PRP to attach to and provide a release of PRP growth factors.[25,26] This material is derived from porcine basement membrane bladder and is a collagen matrix. Although there may be growth factors attached to the material, it is unclear if the factors are active.

Adverse reactions with PRP are uncommon. Sometimes patients complain of a burning sensation for a brief time and localized erythema. Infection is a possibility and there is a reported case of a stroke when PRP was combined with stem cells. The PRP in this instance was being used in a facial cosmetic procedure.[27]

We have found PRP useful in the treatment of alopecia areata. It can be used to enhance vascular neogenesis in areas of scar tissue and provide a more fertile area for subsequent hair transplant surgery. This is very helpful in cases of scalp scarring with atrophic areas.

Porcine Bladder Matrix

Acell is a bio material derived from porcine bladder. It is composed primarily of collagen, elastin, laminin, and fibronectin. There are growth factors inherent to the material but it is unclear as to whether these factors are active when the material is used. The material comes in sheets or in a powder.

Some physicians have used it for the linear scars of strip harvesting, as it is felt that the resultant scar is softer. It is being used for FUE wounds and it may aid in promoting the healing of the wounds as well as stimulating regrowth of new hairs. It is felt that it may stimulate the hair stem cell population and new hairs may arise in the FUE wounds.

Acell is also being combined with PRP in the hopes that the material will provide a scaffold for the PRP and aid in the slow distribution of growth factors from the PRP.

Lasers

Mester originally demonstrated that lasers can aid in wound healing and at a wavelength of 694 aided

in hair growth in mice.[28,29] Over the past decade, it has become evident that low-level lasers can provide a positive effect on human hair growth.[30–33] The mechanism of action is believed to relate to upregulation of cyclic adenosine monophosphate and cyclic guanosine monophosphate. Various cytokines and proteins may be produced that can improve hair growth as well. The use of lasers allows hairs to enter into the anagen phase of hair growth and the hairs tend to stay in anagen longer. The efficacy of the low-level lasers is believed to be similar to that of minoxidil.

Numerous versions of the low-level laser therapy devices exist. Some devices are constructed as a hat, others are a comb or brush or a headband embedded with the light-emitting diodes. Larger units are often used postoperatively to aid in healing and perhaps encourage hair growth.

It remains unclear as to what is the optimal wavelength for hair loss treatment. Additionally, there is no well-developed protocol for usage for this indication thus far. Questions such as to how often the laser should be used, what power should be used, how long should a treatment be, and if there is an inhibitory effect that occurs with overuse, remain unanswered.

Currently, most devices are used a wavelength of 635 to 650 nm. Usage is recommended as 2 to 3 times weekly for 20 to 30 minutes.

Stem Cells

An especially intriguing area of hair transplantation is the use of stem cells. The public has been fascinated with the stories of numerous miraculous cures for many diseases with the use of pluripotent stem cells. Although the evidence for such miracle cures is often lacking, there is little doubt that the use of stem cells may provide major advances in treating many diseases and injuries in the future.

In terms of hair restoration, there is a lack of large-scale studies; nevertheless, the studies available indicate promise of hair growth based primarily on mouse and rat cell models.[34,35] Studies on humans are few.

We are currently undertaking a study involving stem cells for hair growth. We have used adipose-derived stem cells to try to promote hair growth in patients with female pattern hair loss and male pattern hair loss. Our results thus far are encouraging. We have observed growth of hair but it is unclear as to how long the effects will persist.

Body Hair

Many patients who undergo hair restoration have marked hair loss and their donor area is insufficient to supply enough hair to cover both the frontal area and crown. For these patients, it may be reasonable to obtain hair from other locations, such as the beard area or other body areas to try to provide donor hair. Some patients may have areas of hair loss on their face or body where the use of body hair would be ideal for restoring the hair pattern in the area such as the beard area or eyebrows.[36,37]

Body hairs also may be used to refine hair lines and conceal an unacceptable scar. Such grafts have been used in cases in which a scar from strip surgery needs to be improved.[38]

The surgeon must be cognizant of the fact that body hair essentially retains the characteristics of body hair and does not grow like scalp hair. Also, the caliber and wave or curl of the hair may be different from that of the surrounding hair and the patient and physician should discuss how this may impact the aesthetic outcome of the procedure.

Strip surgery can be used to obtain beard hair by incising an ellipse in the area under the chin. This can heal particularly well and provide sufficient grafts for small cases, but most commonly the FUE/FIT (Follicular Isolation Technique) technique is used to obtain beard hair or body hair grafts.

Umar[39] stressed that the surgeon should attempt to obtain hairs that are clearly in the anagen phase of growth. He suggests having patients use 5% minoxidil twice daily for 6 weeks to 6 months before surgery. At 7 to 10 days before surgery, he shaves the donor area to better identify the anagen hairs.

Patients need to be advised that body hair tends to have a lower survival than scalp hair, and many body FUs are single hairs. It is unclear as to why the rate of survival is less. Also, hypopigmented round scars will often be evident from the harvesting of body hairs. The skin in these areas will not generally tan when exposed to sunlight.

Scalp Micropigmentation

Many patients who undergo hair restoration have extensive hair loss. The donor area is limited and therefore it is unlikely that they can adequately transplant the entire area of hair loss. A possible solution to the situation is the use of scalp micropigmentation.[40] Using scalp micropigmentation, the area can be tattooed to provide a sense of coverage. The technique works particularly well for patients that have some hair in the area.

Scalp micropigmentation (SMP) also can be used in patients with traumatic hair loss and scars. SMP has worked particularly well for the linear scars of strip harvesting.[41] Some forms of hair loss from scarring alopecia are also well suited for SMP.

The SMP technique requires special inks and instrumentation. This is not a procedure to be done by the local tattoo artist. A high degree of proficiency is required for an optimal outcome. Needle depth is crucial and proper selection and deposition of the pigment is required to avoid blurring of color and making marks that are too large. If the color is placed too deep, there can be alteration in the apparent color of the pigmentation. This can be very disconcerting for the patient and physician.

SUMMARY

As one might expect, the hair transplant procedure that was once somewhat primitive has become more refined. The surgical technique has become more sophisticated and allows for better use of donor hair, enhanced implantation, and ultimately better cosmetic results.

The recognition of many of the physiologic and genetic aspects of hair development and hair growth has prompted the use of bio-enhancements ranging from storage media to the use of lasers. These additions have aided in graft survival and growth.

As we understand more about the cellular controls of hair loss and hair growth we may be able to provide patients with the "full head" of hair that they want. In the future, our ability to manipulate genetic signals and genes may simply allow us to overcome the genetic signals that cause various forms of hair loss.

REFERENCES

1. Headington JT. Transverse microscopic anatomy of the human scalp. A basis for a morphometric approach to disorders of the hair follicle. Arch Dermatol 1984;120(4):449–56.
2. Bicknell LM, Kash N, Kavouspour C, et al. Follicular unit extraction hair transplant harvest: a review of current recommendations and future considerations. Dermatol Online J 2014;20(3).
3. Rose PT, Nusbaum B. Robotic hair restoration. Dermatol Clin 2014;32(1):97–107.
4. Tykocinski A. Dealing with a hybrid punch. Hair Transplant Forum Int'l 2017;27(1):14–6. Available at: http://www.ishrs.org/content/dealing-hybrid-trumpet-punch. Accessed October 24, 2017.
5. Harris J. Go with Blunt Rotation. Presented at FUE Immersion Course. Polanica Zdroj, Poland, October 1–2, 2017.
6. Rose P. A Novel Punch for FIT. Presented at the ISHRS annual meeting. Las Vegas (NV), September 25–30, 2007.

7. Boaventura O. Long Hair FUE and the Donor Area Preview. Hair Transplant Forum International. 26 September–5 October, 2016.
8. Park JP. Presented at FUE mini course. ISHRS annual meeting. Las Vegas (NV), September 28–October 1, 2016.
9. Choi YC, Kim JC. Single hair transplantation using the Choi hair transplanter. J Dermatol Surg Oncol 1992;18(11):945–8.
10. Park JH. Graft Implanters. In: Unger W, Shapiro R, Unger R, editors. Hair Transplantation, 5th Edition. London: Informa Healthcare; 2011. p. 404–6.
11. Park JH. Novel Implanter technique that enables more than 1600 grafts in one hour with dense packing. ISHRS video library. 2013.
12. Speranzini M. Graft placement using the Dull Needle Implanter Technique. In Hair Transplant Forum International. February 1–23, 2013.
13. Mathew A. A review of cellular bio-preservation considerations during hair transplantation. In Hair Transplant Forum Int'l. January 23– February 1, 2013.
14. Cooley J. Bio-enhanced hair restoration. In Hair Transplant Forum Int'l. 24 July–4 August, 2014.
15. Lacci KM, Dardik A. Platelet-rich plasma: support for its use in wound healing. Yale J Biol Med 2010;83(1):1–9.
16. Reese R. Regenerative medicine part 2: use of platelet rich plasma in hair. In: Lam S, editor. Hair transplant 360. New Delhi (India): Jaypee Brothers Publishing; 2014. p. 565–73.
17. Uebel C. A New Advance in baldness surgery using platelet derived growth factor. Hair Transplant Forum Int'l 2005;15(3):77–84.
18. Gentile P, Garcovich S, Bielli A, et al. The effect of platelet-rich plasma in hair regrowth: a randomized placebo-controlled trial. Stem Cells Transl Med 2015;4(11):1317–23.
19. Li ZJ, Choi HI, Choi DK, et al. Autologous platelet-rich plasma: a potential therapeutic tool for promoting hair growth. Dermatol Surg 2012;38(7 Pt 1):1040–6.
20. Puig CJ, Reese R, Peters M. Double-blind, placebo-controlled pilot study on the use of platelet-rich plasma in women with female androgenetic alopecia. Dermatol Surg 2016;42(11):1243–7.
21. Singh B, Goldberg LJ. Autologous platelet-rich plasma for the treatment of pattern hair loss. Am J Clin Dermatol 2016;17(4):359–67.
22. Yano K, Brown LF, Detmar M. Control of hair growth and follicle size by VEGF-mediated angiogenesis. J Clin Invest 2001;107(4):409–17.
23. Greco J, Brandt R. Preliminary experience and extended applications for the use of autologous platelet rich plasma in hair transplantation surgery. Hair Transplant Forum Int'l 2007;17(4):131–2.
24. Berti AF, Santillan A, Garcia-Corrochano P. Acute stroke after scalp injection of platelet rich plasma and stem cells for hair loss. J Neurol Stroke 2015;3(6).
25. Mester E, Szende B, Gartner P. The effect of laser beams on the growth of hair in mice. Radiobiol Radiother (Berl) 1968;9(5):621–6 [in German].
26. Leavitt M, Charles G, Heyman E, et al. HairMax lasercomb laser phototherapy device in the treatment of male androgenetic alopecia: a randomized, double-blind, sham device-controlled, multicentre trial. Clin Drug Investig 2009;29(5):283–92.
27. Jimenez JJ, Charles G, Heyman E, et al. Efficacy and safety of a low-level laser device in the treatment of male and female pattern hair loss: a multicenter, randomized, sham device-controlled, double-blind study. Am J Clin Dermatol 2014;15(2):115–27.
28. Keene S. The science of light bio-stimulation and low level laser therapy. Hair Transplant Forum Int'l 2014;24(6):208–9.
29. Hamblin M. Mechanism of laser induced hair regrowth, in Wellman Center for Photomedicine. 2006. p. 28–33.
30. Umar S. Use of body hair and beard hair in hair restoration. Facial Plast Surg Clin North Am 2013;21(3):469–77.
31. Toyoshima KE, Asakawa K, Ishibashi N, et al. Fully functional hair follicle regeneration through the rearrangement of stem cells and their niches. Nat Commun 2012;3:784.
32. Nusbaum AG, Rose PT, Nusbaum BP. Nonsurgical therapy for hair loss. Facial Plast Surg Clin North Am 2013;21(3):335–42.
33. Festa E, Fretz J, Berry R, et al. Adipocyte lineage cells contribute to the skin stem cell niche to drive hair cycling. Cell 2011;146(5):761–71.
34. Umar S. Hair transplantation in patients with inadequate head donor supply using nonhead hair: report of 3 cases. Ann Plast Surg 2011;67(4):332–5.
35. Jones R. Body hair transplant into wide donor scar. Dermatol Surg 2008;34(6):857.
36. Park JH, Moh JS, Lee SY, et al. Micropigmentation: camouflaging scalp alopecia and scars in Korean patients. Aesthetic Plast Surg 2014;38(1):199–204.
37. Cooley J. Use of porcine bladder matrix in hair restoration surgery applications. Hair Transplant Forum Int'l 2011;3:70–2.
38. Cole J. Body to scalp hair transplantation. In: Unger W, Shapiro R, Unger R, editors. Hair Transplantation. Hair Transplantation 5th Edition. London: Informa Healthcare; 2011. p. 304–6.
39. Umar S. Body hair transplant by follicular unit extraction: my experience with 122 patients. Aesthet Surg J 2016;36(10):1101–10.
40. Rassman WR, Pak JP, Kim J. Scalp micropigmentation: a useful treatment for hair loss. Facial Plast Surg Clin North Am 2013;21(3):497–503.
41. Traquina AC. Micropigmentation as an adjuvant in cosmetic surgery of the scalp. Dermatol Surg 2001;27(2):123–8.

New-Generation Therapies for the Treatment of Hair Loss in Men

Neil S. Sadick, MD[a,b,*]

KEYWORDS

- PRP • Nutraceuticals • LLLT • Small molecule inhibitors

KEY POINTS

- Selection of hair transplantation methodology depends on patients' goals, type of hair loss, and quality of hair.
- Robotic hair transplantation is the latest frontier in hair restoration.
- Platelet-rich plasma, low-level laser therapy, and stem cells can be used together with hair transplantation to enhance graft survival.

INTRODUCTION

Androgenetic alopecia (AGA), also known as androgenic alopecia or male pattern baldness, is the most common type of progressive hair loss. AGA is less common in Asians, and African Americans are 4 times less likely than whites to develop it. The condition is characterized by the progressive loss of terminal hairs on the scalp in a characteristic distribution with the anterior, mid, temporal, and vertex the typical sites of involvement.[1–4] Aside from physical appearance, hair loss has great impact on psychological well-being and quality of life, with low-esteem, depression, and social anxiety commonly reported.[5] In AGA there is progressive miniaturization of the hair follicle leading to vellus transformation of terminal hair resulting from an alteration in hair cycle dynamics: anagen duration gradually decreases and telogen increases. Although androgens are known to be implicated in these changes, the pathophysiology driving hair loss is still largely unknown. Current scientific data support that hair loss is likely a multifactorial disorder caused by interactions among several genes and intrinsic/extrinsic environmental factors.

Genetics play an important role in male AGA. As 1 study showed in 500 monozygotic and 400 dizygotic male twins between the ages of 25 and 36, 80% of the variance in the extent of hair loss was attributed to genetic effects.[6] Numerous studies have identified genetic susceptibility loci for AGA, including the androgen receptor/EDAR2 locus on the X chromosome.[7] Exposure to UV light, smoking, pollutants, poor nutrition, and other factors have also been shown to lead to the production of reactive oxygen species and release of proinflammatory cytokines, leading to a state of inflammation and oxidative stress that contributes to hair loss. Evidence of the causative role of inflammation in driving hair loss was highlighted in a study by Sadick and colleagues that included 52 female subjects with AGA, with superficial lymphocytic perifolliculitis involving the superficial isthmic part of the follicle. Treatment of the subjects with anti-inflammatory medications together with minoxidil was more efficacious clinically than monotherapy alone, implying that the

Disclosure Statement: N. Sadick has nothing to disclose.
[a] Department of Dermatology, Weill Cornell Medicine, New York, NY, USA; [b] Department of Dermatology, University of Buffalo, Buffalo, NY, USA
* 911 Park Avenue, New York, NY 10075.
E-mail address: nssderm@sadickdermatology.com

Dermatol Clin 36 (2018) 63–67
http://dx.doi.org/10.1016/j.det.2017.08.003
0733-8635/18/© 2017 Elsevier Inc. All rights reserved.

inflammatory process is key to perpetuating disordered hair physiology.[8] Chronically elevated psychoemotional stress is also increasingly recognized as contributing to hair loss through to the production of stress hormones, like cortisol, which are known to induce catagen.[9]

In terms of current treatment, the 2 therapeutic agents approved by the Food and Drug Administration and European Medicines Agency for treatment of AGA are topical minoxidil and oral finasteride (1 mg/d).[10] Both these agents, however, have had a limited success rate, and, even worse, unfavorable side effects, including sexual dysfunction. More importantly, these therapies fail to address the complex pathophysiology driving hair loss and rely on targeting singular compounds androgens (finasteride) rather than considering a more comprehensive approach that targets stress and inflammation. New therapies, such as PRP, injectable cytokines, low-level laser therapy (LLLT), and nutraceuticals are emerging with promising results, testament to the validity of a paradigm shift in hair loss treatments, one that recognizes and addresses the complexity of hair loss biology.

PLATELET-RICH PLASMA

Platelet-rich plasma (PRP) injections have been used for some time in several medical fields, such as in regenerative medicine, sport medicine, and aesthetic dermatology/plastic surgery.[11] In the past couple years, several lines of investigation have reported positive results in the use of PRP for treatment of hair loss. Compared with drugs, PRP injections are safe and cheap, without major side effects, and require only periodic treatment sessions.[12] This is an attractive alternative for patients who have tried finasteride and experienced undesirable side effects or do not want the long-term commitment necessary for minoxidil application. PRP is ideal for mild/moderate hair loss as monotherapy or adjuvant to other procedures, such as hair transplantation.

PRP is an autologous product that is manufactured by centrifugation from patients' own venous blood, limiting the potential risk of disease transmission. Its utility in the treatment of androgenic alopecia is rooted in the presence of growth factors in plasma factors that are important for cell proliferation and differentiation and has anti-inflammatory properties. The main growth factors are platelet-derived growth factor (PDGF), transforming growth factor (TGF)-β1 and TGF-β2, vascular endothelial growth factor (VEGF), basic fibroblastic growth factor , epidemic growth factor, insulinlike growth factors (IGF-1, IGF-2,

and IGF-3), and hepatocyte growth factor (HGF).[13,14] The mechanism via which PRP is proposed to stimulate hair growth is through the promotion of vascularization and angiogenesis as well as the entry and extension of the duration of the anagen phase of the hair cycle.[15] This is achieved by growth factor–mediated increased activation of wingless (Wnt)/β-catenin, extracellular signal–regulated kinase (ERK), and protein kinase B (Akt) signaling pathways, which lead to cellular proliferation and differentiation in the hair follicle.[16]

Although there is a need for larger, more controlled clinical trials with longer follow-up periods and standardized protocols and dose regimes, a recent meta-analysis summarizing PRP studies thus far has shown the treatment overall results in quantitatively beneficial outcomes.[17] In 177 patients treated with PRP, significantly locally increased hair numbers per square centimeter were observed after PRP injections versus control along with a significantly increased hair thickness cross-section per 10^4 square millimeters favoring the PRP group.

INJECTABLE CYTOKINES

Another hair treatment modality currently in development and similar to PRP in terms of its lack of side effects and dosing but not autologous is injectable cytokines, offered by Histogen (San Diego, California) and marketed as Hair Stimulating Complex (HSC). HSC is a soluble injectable formulation based on cell conditioned media (CCM) produced by neonatal cells grown in suspension under simulated embryonic conditions of hypoxia (3%–5% oxygen). Under these conditions, cells become multipotent and secrete key growth factors including keratinocyte growth factor (KGF), VEGF, and follistatin, which have been linked to hair follicle stem cell proliferation. Two proof-of-concept clinical trials of an earlier prototype of CCM were completed outside the United States, reveal promising efficacy results.[18] In 1 trial, 84.6% of patients receiving just 1 treatment showed a significant increase in terminal hair count and hair thickness at 12 weeks and results were sustained at the 12-month follow-up. In the second clinical trial, in which patients received 2 treatments 6 weeks apart, the increase in total hair count was 46.5% above that seen after a single treatment. Significant improvements were observed in total hair count, terminal hairs, and hair thickness at 12 weeks and 1 year. After these initial studies, Histogen plans to conduct a phase 1 clinical study in the United States using HSC, which is purified to enrich for KGF, VEGF, follistatin, and additional growth factors known to be necessary for hair growth: placental growth factor, angiogenin, and HGF.

LOW-LEVEL LASER THERAPY

LLLT, also called red light therapy, bio-stimulation, and photobiomodulation, is a safe form of light/heat treatment evaluated for a variety of medical conditions, including acne, skin rejuvenation, fat reduction, and more recently hair loss. LLLT is thought to promote tissue repair and regeneration by stimulating cellular activity when penetrating through the scalp.[19] The most commonly used wavelengths are in the range of 500 nm to 1100 nm and deliver fluences of 1 J/cm^2 to 10 J/cm^2 with a power density of 3 mW/cm^2 to 90 mW/cm^2.[20] LLLT devices are available either as in-office hoods or overhead panels bonnet or at-home head caps/helmets/combs. Treatment protocols vary but according to the author's experience, in-office treatment protocols that are efficacious involve 1 weekly 30-minute treatment for 8 weeks and 1 bimonthly treatment for another 8 weeks, followed by 1 treatment twice a year and quarterly treatments for maintenance. At-home hair growth devices are also useful when used devices for 20 minutes, 2 times to 3 times a week.

Although the exact LLLT mechanism of action is unclear, evidence suggests that LLLT, by stimulating the mitochondrial cell metabolism, releases nitric oxide from cytochrome c oxidase, leading to increased ATP production, decreased oxidative stress, and thus reduced free reactive oxygen species levels and induction of cell proliferation signaling, such as nuclear factor κB. These events result in improved circulation; decreased inflammation; stimulation of hair follicle growth due to the presence of growth factors, such as HGF, VEGF, and IGF-1; and decreased levels of catagen-inducing dihydrotestosterone (DHT).[21,22]

Most studies investigating effects of LLLT on hair growth have used wavelengths that range from 635 nm to 650 nm, but near-infrared wavelengths, such as 810 nm, which have deeper penetrating capacities, have also been used.[23] A recent study comparing the effectiveness of a 665-nm low-level diode laser hat versus a combination of 665-nm and 808-nm low-level diode laser scanners on hair growth in AGA showed a statistically significant improvement in hair growth for the combination treatment group compared with the laser hat and control group alone.[24] A meta-analysis assessing the efficacy of nonsurgical treatments of AGA (minoxidil, finasteride, and LLLT) in comparison with placebo for improving hair density, thickness, and growth demonstrated that LLLT was effective for promoting hair growth in men with AGA with no side effects.[25]

NUTRACEUTICALS

Several nutraceuticals have also emerged and have been studied for their potential hair growth benefits. These are products derived from food sources that are purported to provide extra health benefits, such as prevention of chronic disease and aging, in addition to the basic nutritional value found in foods. Nutraceutical ingredients are mostly constituted by botanicals that have pleio-tropic biological effects and are able to target several cellular pathways at once. Although the mechanism of action of these formulations is not known, it is hypothesized that cumulating ingredients with antioxidant, anti-inflammatory, and cell proliferative ingredients has synergistic effects in promoting hair growth and reducing cellular damage at the level of the hair follicle.

One of the first nutraceuticals for hair loss was Viviscal (Lifes2good, Chicago, Illinois), incorporating special marine extracts and a silica compound. An early randomized, double-blind, study comparing the effects of Viviscal with those of a fish extract for the treatment of AGA showed that twice-daily intake of the supplement for 6 months led to a statistically significant increase in nonvellus hair of 38% of patients receiving Viviscal compared with a 2% increase in the fish extract treatment group. Moreover 95% of the Viviscal subjects showed both clinical and histologic cure at the end of treatment whereas none of the subjects treated with fish extract showed any clinical or histologic difference in the same timeframe.[26] A new-generation formulation of Viviscal, containing marine complex, biotin, vitamin C, and apple extract, was also shown in a recent 6-month, randomized, double-blind, placebo-controlled study to promote hair growth in men with AGA.[27]

Another supplement, Forti5 (Q-SkinScience, Miami, FL), containing green tea extract, omega-3 and omega-6 fatty acids, cholecalciferol, melatonin, β-sitosterol, and soy isoflavones, was shown in a proof-of-concept clinical trial to benefit hair growth: after 24 weeks of twice-daily supplements, 80% of subjects had improved hair count, with 40% rating it moderate and 10% rating is great.[28]

Nutrafol is another new nutraceutical supplement on the market that selectively uses patented, bio-optimized botanic ingredients that have clinical data on absorption and efficacy and are standardized to contain consistent fractions of phytoactive components. Key ingredients of Nutrafol are curcumin, ashwagandha, saw palmetto, vitamin E, and 17 more ingredients, including minerals, resveratrol, horsetail, marine collagen, and hyaluronic acid. The supplement was designed to target the multiple underlying causes of hair loss, particularly on relatively new aspects like inflammation, stress, and oxidative damage, in addition to more well-studied parameters like DHT.

Currently 3 randomized, placebo-controlled, double-blind trials are in progress, to evaluate the clinical safety and efficacy of Nutrafol, while several case series and physician reports have demonstrated promising results in treating hair loss either as monotherapy or in combination with other modalities like PRP.

MICRONEEDLING AND ENERGY-BASED DEVICES

Scalp microneedling and energy-based devices, such as fractional lasers/radiofrequency, have also been explored in their ability to promote hair growth. These strategies have been documented as effective in several dermatologic conditions, such as acne scars, skin rejuvenation by creating microinjuries and subsequently stimulating a wound-healing response. The proposed mechanism of action of these treatments includes up-regulation of hair-related genes, release of growth factors (PDGF and VEGF), and activation of follicle stem cells.[29-31]

A 12-week randomized, evaluator-blinded study in 100 patients with mild to moderate AGA comparing weekly microneedling treatment, combined with 5% topical minoxidil twice daily, to only 5% topical minoxidil twice daily showed that the mean hair count was significantly higher in the microneedling group.[30] A follow-up case series in 4 men (already taking finasteride and minoxidil) who received 4 weekly microneedling sessions followed by 11 sessions at 2-week intervals, for a total of 24 weeks of treatment, showed high patient satisfaction from all subjects and results were maintained at the 18-month postprocedure follow-up.[29]

Although microneedling/energy devices seem to be a promising hair treatment, there is a paucity of studies using this modality as monotherapy; thus, more studies are needed to standardize treatment protocols and document their safety and efficacy. In the author's experience, microneedling and energy-based devices deliver synergistic effects when used in combination with PRP, LLLT, and conventional drugs, and clinical trials are under way to evaluate the optimal combination strategies.

SUMMARY

Treatment of AGA is an extremely challenging feat for the medical community, given the complex biology of hair, and the interplay of intrinsic/extrinsic factors that drive the pathophysiology of hair loss. A promising step toward hair loss treatment is the design of therapeutics that do not target 1 aspect of hair loss, such as hormones, but comprehensively address and target all hair loss triggers. Continued evaluation of the new treatments described (PRP, LLLT, and nutraceuticals) in the clinic should be performed to establish their efficacy and safety and optimize therapeutic protocols to ensure successful clinical outcomes.

REFERENCES

1. Hamilton JB. Patterned loss of hair in man; types and incidence. Ann N Y Acad Sci 1951; 53(3):708–28.
2. Levy-Nissenbaum E, Bar-Natan M, Frydman M, et al. Confirmation of the association between male pattern baldness and the androgen receptor gene. Eur J Dermatol 2005;15(5):339–40.
3. Otberg N, Finner AM, Shapiro J. Androgenetic alopecia. Endocrinol Metab Clin North Am 2007;36(2): 379–98.
4. Schweiger ES, Boychenko O, Bernstein RM. Update on the pathogenesis, genetics and medical treatment of patterned hair loss. J Drugs Dermatol 2010;9(11):1412–9.
5. Wells PA, Willmoth T, Russell RJ. Does fortune favour the bald? Psychological correlates of hair loss in males. Br J Psychol 1995;86(Pt 3):337–44.
6. Nyholt DR, Gillespie NA, Heath AC, et al. Genetic basis of male pattern baldness. J Invest Dermatol 2003;121(6):1561–4.
7. Hillmer AM, Hanneken S, Ritzmann S, et al. Genetic variation in the human androgen receptor gene is the major determinant of common early-onset androgenetic alopecia. Am J Hum Genet 2005; 77(1):140–8.
8. Magro CM, Rossi A, Poe J, et al. The role of inflammation and immunity in the pathogenesis of androgenetic alopecia. J Drugs Dermatol 2011;10(12): 1404–11.
9. Peters EM, Liotiri S, Bodó E, et al. Probing the effects of stress mediators on the human hair follicle: substance P holds central position. Am J Pathol 2007;171(6):1872–86.
10. Kelly Y, Blanco A, Tosti A. Androgenetic alopecia: an update of treatment options. Drugs 2016;76(14): 1349–64.
11. Sommeling CE, Heyneman A, Hoeksema H, et al. The use of platelet-rich plasma in plastic surgery: a systematic review. J Plast Reconstr Aesthet Surg 2013;66(3):301–11.
12. Li ZJ, Choi HI, Choi DK, et al. Autologous platelet-rich plasma: a potential therapeutic tool for

promoting hair growth. Dermatol Surg 2012; 38(7 Pt 1):1040–6.

13. Eppley BL, Woodell JE, Higgins J. Platelet quantification and growth factor analysis from platelet-rich plasma: implications for wound healing. Plast Reconstr Surg 2004;114(6):1502–8.

14. Miao Y, Sun YB, Sun XJ, et al. Promotional effect of platelet-rich plasma on hair follicle reconstitution in vivo. Dermatol Surg 2013;39(12):1868–76.

15. Ferneini EM, Beauvais D, Castiglione C, et al. Platelet-rich plasma in androgenic alopecia: indications, technique, and potential benefits. J Oral Maxillofac Surg 2017;75(4):788–95.

16. Gupta AK, Carviel J. A mechanistic model of platelet-rich plasma treatment for androgenetic alopecia. Dermatol Surg 2016;42(12):1335–9.

17. Giordano S, Romeo M, Lankinen P. Platelet-rich plasma for androgenetic alopecia: does it work? Evidence from meta analysis. J Cosmet Dermatol 2017;16(3):374–81.

18. Zimber MP, Ziering C, Zeigler F, et al. Hair regrowth following a Wnt- and follistatin containing treatment: safety and efficacy in a first-in-man phase 1 clinical trial. J Drugs Dermatol 2011;10(11):1308–12.

19. Schindl A, Schindl M, Pernerstorfer-Schön H, et al. Low-intensity laser therapy: a review. J Investig Med 2000;48(5):312–26.

20. Avci P, Gupta GK, Clark J, et al. Low-level laser (light) therapy (LLLT) for treatment of hair loss. Lasers Surg Med 2014;46(2):144–51.

21. Chung H, Dai T, Sharma SK, et al. The nuts and bolts of low-level laser (light) therapy. Ann Biomed Eng 2012;40(2):516–33.

22. Lohr NL, Keszler A, Pratt P, et al. Enhancement of nitric oxide release from nitrosyl hemoglobin and nitrosyl myoglobin by red/near infrared radiation: potential role in cardioprotection. J Mol Cell Cardiol 2009;47(2):256–63.

23. Kim TH, Kim NJ, Youn JI. Evaluation of wavelength-dependent hair growth effects on low-level laser therapy: an experimental animal study. Lasers Med Sci 2015;30(6):1703–9.

24. Barikbin B, Khodamrdi Z, Kholoosi L, et al. Comparison of the effects of 665 nm low level diode laser hat versus and a combination of 665 nm and 808nm low level diode laser scanner of hair growth in androgenic alopecia. J Cosmet Laser Ther 2017. [Epub ahead of print].

25. Adil A, Godwin M. The effectiveness of treatments for androgenetic alopecia: a systematic review and meta-analysis. J Am Acad Dermatol 2017;77(1):136–41.e5.

26. Lassus A, Eskelinen E. A comparative study of a new food supplement, ViviScal, with fish extract for the treatment of hereditary androgenic alopecia in young males. J Int Med Res 1992;20(6):445–53.

27. Ablon G. A 6-month, randomized, double-blind, placebo-controlled study evaluating the ability of a marine complex supplement to promote hair growth in men with thinning hair. J Cosmet Dermatol 2016;15(4):358–66.

28. Nichols AJ, Hughes OB, Canazza A, et al. An open-label evaluator blinded study of the efficacy and safety of a new nutritional supplement in androgenetic alopecia: a pilot study. J Clin Aesthet Dermatol 2017;10(2):52–6.

29. Dhurat R, Mathapati S. Response to microneedling treatment in men with androgenetic alopecia who failed to respond to conventional therapy. Indian J Dermatol 2015;60(3):260–3.

30. Dhurat R, Sukesh M, Avhad G, et al. A randomized evaluator blinded study of effect of microneedling in androgenetic alopecia: a pilot study. Int J Trichology 2013;5(1):6–11.

31. Kim YS, Jeong KH, Kim JE, et al. Repeated microneedle stimulation induces enhanced hair growth in a murine model. Ann Dermatol 2016;28(5):586–92.

Combination Therapy for Male Cosmetic Patients

Michael H. Gold, MD[a,b,c,d,e,f,g,h,i,j],*

KEYWORDS

- Combination therapy • Male patients • Cosmetic procedures

KEY POINTS

- Combination therapy for cosmetic procedures for men is an important consideration to give optimal outcomes to men with cosmetic concerns.
- More evidence-based medicine is needed to document that the combination works, that it is safe, and that the end result is what we are looking to achieve.
- When done correctly, men will be more likely to request advice on how to enhance their cosmetic appearance.

INTRODUCTION

Men have as many cosmetic concerns as their female counterparts, yet we see more women in our clinics. This circumstance is due to a variety of reasons; but regardless, we seem to be reaching more and more men in the cosmetic arena than ever before as we end 2017 and begin 2018. Increasing numbers of nonsurgical cosmetic procedures are being performed on men, which is beneficial to both the patients and the cosmetic surgeons.

Since the economic downturn and eventual recovery of the past decade, more and more men, either active or entering the market place, realize that their physical appearance is important when presenting themselves to potential employers or clients. For these reasons, most of us have seen an increase in the number of men that seek cosmetic procedures; many of these procedures entail using combination therapy for optimal results. The most common of the cosmetic nonsurgical cosmetic procedures performed on men, according to the American Society for Aesthetic Plastic Surgeons (ASAPS) are intense pulsed light (IPL) treatments (13.9% men), laser hair removal (12.9% men,) and neurotoxin injections (11.5% men).[1,2]

This article reviews the most common male cosmetic procedures that are performed in combination with more than one procedure. Evidence-based medicine for many of these combination therapies is not rampant in the medical literature, but the author uses his current experience to share how combining therapies can be useful for the male population seeking cosmetic improvements in our offices.

Disclosure: The author has nothing to disclose.
[a] Gold Skin Care Center, Tennessee Clinical Research Center, 2000 Richard Jones Road, Suite 220, Nashville, TN 37215, USA; [b] Vanderbilt University School of Nursing, Nashville, TN, USA; [c] Meharry Medical College, School of Medicine, Nashville, TN, USA; [d] Wake Forest School of Medicine, Winston-Salem, NC, USA; [e] Huashan Hospital, Fudan University, Shanghai, China; [f] First Hospital of China Medical University, Shenyang, China; [g] Guangdong Provincial People's Hospital, Guangzhou, China; [h] First People's Hospital of Foshan, Guangzhou, China; [i] Zhejiang University, Hangzhou, Zhejiang, China; [j] Rongjun Hospital, Jiaxing, China
* Gold Skin Care Center, Tennessee Clinical Research Center, 2000 Richard Jones Road, Suite 220, Nashville, TN 37215.
E-mail address: drgold@goldskincare.com

Nonsurgical cosmetic procedures have been described in detail elsewhere in this supplement; thus, the author's focus is on using a combination approach to therapy. Combination treatments provide perhaps the best aesthetic outcomes, which are described in this article. How do we use neurotoxins with dermal fillers? How do we use skin care with everything we do? How do we combine fat reduction with skin tightening? How do we use absorbable sutures with skin tightening? Finally, how do we use platelet-rich plasma (PRP) with hair transplants to enhance the results we now see with our hair transplant procedures?

COMBINATION THERAPIES FOR MEN

The advent and use of botulinum A neurotoxin has been the real game changer for most of us in the cosmetic and aesthetic industry over the past several decades. The author has seen the number of procedures from the statistics of both the ASAPS and the American Society for Dermatologic Surgery (ASDS). Both of these groups have shown that the number of these procedures has been steadily increasing, and they are the most common nonsurgical cosmetic procedures that are performed in our offices over this period in total. There has been an increase in the growth rate of these neurotoxin injections in men; according to the statistics given, the use of neurotoxin injections has increased from 9.2% of all nonsurgical cosmetic procedures performed on men in 2005 to 11.5% of nonsurgical cosmetic procedures performed on men in 2014, according to data from the ASAPS. According to the ASDS, the number of neurotoxin injections performed on men was 10% of all procedures in 2011 and increased to 13% in 2014.[1] The use of Botox Cosmetic (Allergan, Irvine, CA), Dysport (Galderma, For Worth, TX), and Xeomin (Merz Aesthetics, Raleigh, NC) have all transformed our approach to the aesthetic market and to our patients with lines and wrinkles that concern them. This point is true for both women and men. We need to make sure that we consider the potential differences in anatomy and muscle size in men; men may require more neurotoxin than women when giving these injections for the same indications. But with skill and an understanding of the anatomy of the face in both women and men, success with injections for both can be successfully achieved.

Although on most occasions these injections are given without other procedures being performed at the same time, the author always recommends that men, who are less likely to use skin care, incorporate a skin care routine with these injections to enhance the results given and to provide adequate skin protection following the investment that one is taking with these and any cosmetic procedure. And when one talks of skin care, we must always recommend sunscreens to our patients, the most important skin care group we have and something the author tries to make sure male patients are using on a daily basis. Also, as has been shown, the use of neurotoxins and IPL has been shown to improve and enhance the results of using a neurotoxin alone. So, in many instances, where an IPL is indicated, the author often recommends having the IPL treatments given along with the neurotoxin injection. And if there are other concerns, such as wrinkles, telangiectasias, and flushing, the use of neurotoxins given in a mesotherapy approach has been shown to be a very useful combination treatment, something that would benefit men as well as women.[3]

Soft tissue dermal fillers are also a popular cosmetic procedure being performed on more and more men. What has been noted is that the growth rate for these fillers has not changed too significantly as we see with the neurotoxin injections. According to the ASPAS's surveys, the use of dermal fillers was 8.2% of all nonsurgical cosmetic procedures in 2005 and only grew to 8.3% in 2014. The ASDS's data correlates with the ASAPS's data as well, showing an increase from 8% to 9% from 2011 to 2014.[1] This finding may, to some, seem rather surprising; but one can assume from the results presented that neurotoxin procedures are more popular today than ever before and that perhaps clinicians are not recommending dermal fillers as much to our patients when we are evaluating them for wrinkles and lines and, with fillers, for volumization. Many of us had our initial burst of male patients when we had the approval of Sculptra (Galderma, Fort Worth, TX) in our patients with human immunodeficiency virus with lipoatrophy. The author has also, over the years, had great success with all of the hyaluronic acid dermal fillers and volumizers, with the Polly L Lactic Acid product for aesthetic volumization and with calcium hydroxyapatite for wrinkles and contour defects in male patients. But statistically, according to the ASAPS and the ASDS, we are not overall injecting more patients today than we were several years ago.

But when one thinks of combination therapy for our patients, the use of neurotoxins, where appropriate, along with dermal fillers and skin care is, perhaps, the best combination for our male patients to reduce lines and wrinkles, to volumize the skin where appropriate, and, with skin care, to protect and treat any other skin concerns. When appropriate, the use of these products with IPL, or other laser technologies, can improve and enhance the skin as well. Many of the lasers we use every day in our practices can be used in combination without fillers, and many use them regularly.

Fat removal is one of the more popular procedures that are being performed, and there are several current and popular technologies that are being used regularly in our clinics. These technologies include CoolSculpting (Zeltiq, A Division of Allergan, Irvine, CA) and ultrasound devices, such as UltraShape, now known as UltraShape Power (Syneron-Candela, Yokneam, Israel). Alone, they work very well in reducing stubborn areas of fat and have been demonstrated to be safe and efficacious in how they work for patients in this regard. CoolSculpting has become the number one fat reduction treatment in the world and is used on more and more men each and every day. The results of this treatment are well documented and are not reviewed here. What is interesting is that when one combines CoolSculpting with either acoustic wave technology or with radiofrequency (RF) skin tightening, we know that we can achieve even better results than just using CoolSculpting alone. Clinical work with the Z Wave acoustic wave device (Zimmer Aesthetics, Germany) has shown that we can improve the results of our CoolSculpting treatments; this is recommended immediately after most of the CoolSculpting procedures that the author performs.[4] An example of this is shown in **Fig. 1**. In addition, the use of RF skin tightening devices after CoolSculpting treatments has also shown enhancements with the overall cosmetic results. In one study, Few and colleagues[5] described the use of the Venus Legacy (Venus Concepts, Toronto, Canada) and showed it increased efficacy and better cosmetic outcomes following the use of CoolSculpting in a series of patients. Ten patients were evaluated in this clinical protocol and were treated with CoolSculpting and then randomized to receive posttreatment RF treatments versus no further treatment. The results showed a statistically significant improvement on the sides that received the RF therapy as compared with those that did not receive them. An example is shown in **Fig. 2**. From these findings, it seems that if one is performing CoolSculpting in your offices, you ought to be offering either acoustic wave technology or one of the myriad RF skin-tightening devices that exist on the market.

The UltraShape Power is a focused ultrasound device that has been shown to effectively destroy fat cells.[6] One of the things that we all learned early on with this device is that by adding RF skin tightening, one can enhance the results that we had seen with the ultrasound alone. In the US market, the devices that have been improved have been made with only the ultrasound component. Outside the United States, the device marketed

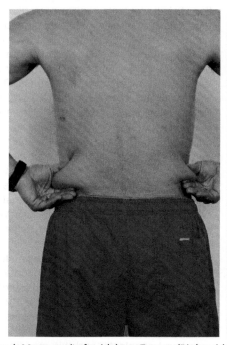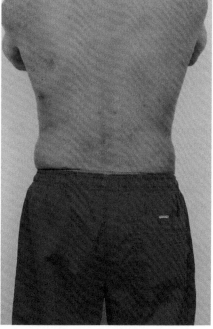

Fig. 1. Hand Massage (Left side) vs Zwave (Right side) Photo taken two months post Cryogenic Lipolysis (Coolsculpting™). Results after one Coolsculpting treatment followed by hand massage on the left and Zwave on the right. (*Photo Courtesy of* John Shieh, MD, RejuvaYou Medical Spa, Pasadena, CA.)

A

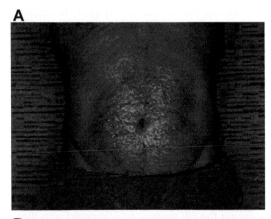

B

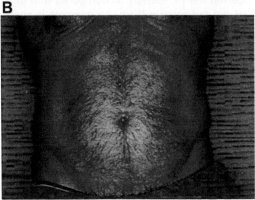

Fig. 2. Male patient at baseline (*A*) and the 6-month follow-up. (*B*) Both flanks were treated with cryolipolisis, but the left flank received additional treatment with multipolar RF/PEMF/suction. (*From* Few J, Gold M, Sadick N, et al. Prospective internally controlled blind reviewed clinical evaluation of cryolipolysis combined with multipolar radiofrequency and varipulse technology for enhanced subject results in circumferential fat reduction and skin laxity of the flanks. J Drugs Dermatol 2016;15(11):1354–8; with permission.)

combines ultrasound with RF energy in one device to make the procedures more efficacious. The new UltraShape Power gives significant energy to have effective fat reduction. But when adding RF, the author does see significantly better clinical results. The author combines the UltraShape Power along with the VelaShape III (Syneron-Candela, Yokneam, Israel) to optimize results. Various protocols have been looked at to determine the best way for this combination to proceed, but the author has not found that one works necessarily better than another. The author does think that pretreatment with the VelaShape III, then using the UltraShape Power, and then resuming skin tightening with the VelaShape III does give patients the best combination and, thus, the best cosmetic outcome.

The Silhouette InstaLift (Sinclair Pharma, London, England) is an absorbable suture technique that is used for lifting the skin and long-term volumization of the skin. In the United States, this suture and associated cone technology is made of both polylactic and polyglycolic acid. Work in the United States has shown that it is a very useful procedure, and recently a consensus article on its use has been published.[7] It is very effective for men and used on the author's male patients who cannot have any associated downtime and want a procedure that takes a relatively short period of time to perform by qualified clinicians. This procedure, combined with ThermiTite (Thermi, an Almirall Company, Dallas, TX), an injectable RF technology, is a wonderful combination to lift and volumize the skin as well as tighten areas, such as the neck. An example of this is shown in **Fig. 3**.

Hair transplants have been a male-dominated cosmetic procedure, although women also benefit greatly from them when needed and when appropriately performed. Hair transplant procedures have progressed recently from what has been known as the donor strip method to more automated systems that remove follicular units of 1 to 2 hairs with minimal to no donor area scars, something that has been a detriment to many who may benefit from a hair transplant but were wary of the potential for noticeable donor site scarring from the strip method of hair transplantation. In addition, hair transplants require a surgeon's artistic touch, as one needs to create an appropriate frontal hair line in most and this needs to be done with care, accuracy, and skill so as to create a normal-appearing frontal hair line. The automated systems, which involve the NeoGraft Hair Transplant System (NeoGraft, Charlotte, NC) and the Artas Robot (Restoration Robotics, San Jose, CA), both use follicular unit extractions to create the follicular units now required to give hair transplant surgeons the best cosmetic outcomes.

PRP has been used more and more in many fields of medicine but has found increasing popularity in the cosmetic arena for a variety of concerns, including those with hair loss looking for an increase in hair growth and in combination with hair transplants to enhance the hair transplant experience. Although many may be skeptical of the use of PRP, as large clinical controlled trials are lacking, there are many reports and case series of successes with the use of PRP for hair growth and as an adjunct to hair transplantation.[8] More and more clinicians are opting to use PRP with hair transplants, and this may be an appropriate combination for one to consider if one is performing this procedure.

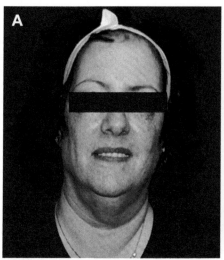
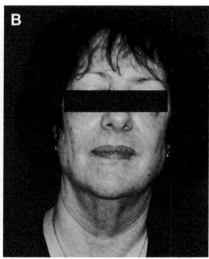

Fig. 3. ThermoTite InstaLift: (*A*) Before treatment and (*B*) 3 months after treatment. (*Courtesy of* Dr Gold, Gold Skin Care Center, The Laser and Rejuvenation Center, Nashville, TN.)

SUMMARY

Combination therapies for cosmetic procedures for men are important considerations for us to give optimal results for the men who come to us for cosmetic concerns. What is needed and seems lacking at this time is more evidence-based medicine for us to use as a source of documentation that the combination works, that it is safe, and achieves the desired results. But when done correctly, more and more men will be coming to our clinics looking for advice on how to enhance their cosmetic concern; we can and will be able to offer them cosmetic and aesthetic procedures that allow them to have the results they are looking for, which then translates, it is hoped, into more self-confidence and self-assurance.

REFERENCES

1. Frucht CS, Ortiz AE. Nonsurgical cosmetic procedures for men: trends and technique considerations. J Clin Aesthet Dermatol 2016;9(12):33–43.
2. Carruthers J, Carruthers A. The effect of full-face broadband light treatments alone and in combination with bilateral crow's feet botulinum toxin type A chemodenervation. Dermatol Surg 2004;30(3):355–66.
3. El Bedewi A. The effect of mesobotox together with intense pulsed light on facial wrinkles and erythema. J Chem Dermatol Sci Appl 2012;2:16–9.
4. Hunt J, Stork H. Cryolipolysis and acoustic wave therapy. Prime 2013;9:112–3.
5. Few J, Gold M, Sadick N. Prospective internally controlled blind reviewed clinical evaluation of cryolipolysis combined with multipolar radiofrequency and varipulse technology for enhanced subject results in circumferential fat reduction and skin laxity of the flanks. J Drugs Dermatol 2016;15(11):1354–8.
6. Coleman WP 3rd, Coleman W 4th, Weiss RA, et al. A multicenter controlled study to evaluate multiple treatments with nonthermal focused ultrasound for noninvasive fat reduction. Dermatol Surg 2017; 43(1):50–7.
7. Nestor MS, Ablon G, Andriessen A, et al. Expert consensus on absorbable advanced suspension technology for facial tissue repositioning and volume enhancement. J Drugs Dermatol 2017;16(7):661–6.
8. Uebal CO, Braga del Silva J, Canterelli D, et al. The role of platelet plasma growth factors in male pattern baldness surgery. Plast Reconstr Surg 2006;118:1458–66.

Liposuction Considerations in Men

Cheryl Karcher, MD[a,b],*

KEYWORDS

- Liposuction • Men • Ultrasound • Laser • Radiofrequency • Fat

KEY POINTS

- Male anatomy and fat distribution are different from the female anatomy.
- The most common areas for male liposuction are breasts, abdomen, flanks, and neck.
- Recovery, complications, and safety of liposuction in men is similar to that in women.

INTRODUCTION

Over the years, the number of men seeking cosmetic interventions has consistently increased by approximately 10% per year. The popularity of treatments such as liposuction are at an all-time high, because it has proven to be, for the right patient, a safe and effective way to reduce fat and improve physique. According to data released by the American Society for Aesthetic Plastic Surgery, Americans spent more than $15 billion during the calendar year on aesthetic cosmetic procedures, and liposuction accounted for 56% of the total expenditures. The top surgical procedure for men was liposuction, with more than 45,012 procedures performed, predominantly in those aged 35 to 50 years.[1]

GENDER CONSIDERATIONS DURING LIPOSUCTION CONSULTATION

During consultation with male patients regarding liposuction, the practicing dermatologist needs to be aware, aside from traditional methodologies (medical history, etc) of the behavioral differences of men compared with women. Both genders have similar goals and expectations regarding the treatment, with fat reduction and body sculpting being the main intentions. Men, however, are more direct in their approach and are more likely to follow through with the procedure after the consultation.

They are generally satisfied with the results, and flaws such as slight asymmetry and irregularities are not distressing to them, as opposed to women, who are more likely to return for correctional surgery and seek perfection. Speedy recovery and simple instructions also fair well with men, because their pain threshold is lower than that of women and they are less compliant with postoperative instructions. Despite the wide acceptance of the male seeking aesthetic treatments in our time, men still prefer to be private and discreet about engaging in a surgical treatment such as liposuction. To this end, liposuction has transformed male body sculpting for men because only small incisions are used, which can by concealed easily or difficult to see. With men, the advantages are seen early on, whereas the downside of treating this population emerges more frequently in the postoperative stage. Men can be better candidates for liposuction than women, because they tend to take fewer medications.[2]

FAT AND LIPOSUCTION TARGET LOCATIONS IN MEN

The subcutaneous fat is distributed anatomically into the apical, mantle, and deep layers. Deep fat is loosely organized and is the main target of liposuction, whereas superficial fat is dense and contained within fibrous bands. The traditional

Disclosure Statement: The author has nothing they wish to disclose.
[a] Department of Dermatology, Weill Cornell Medicine, New York, NY, USA; [b] Sadick Dermatology, 911 Park Avenue, New York, NY 10128, USA
* Sadick Dermatology, 911 Park Avenue, New York, NY 10128, USA
E-mail address: cherylkarcher@yahoo.com

Dermatol Clin 36 (2018) 75–80
https://doi.org/10.1016/j.det.2017.09.010
0733-8635/18/© 2017 Elsevier Inc. All rights reserved.

derm.theclinics.com

liposuction technique consists of deep and subdermal removal of fat and liposculpture can be achieved by careful removal or sculpture of the superficial fat layer. Fat distribution largely depends on genetics, race, and gender.[3] The presence of anabolic hormones such as testosterone results in men having more muscle mass and less superficial fat than women, and metabolic differences between the genders result in different fat distribution in the body. Women accumulate more fat in the thighs, hips, and buttocks, whereas men tend to have more fat in the abdomen, trunk, and chin/neck region. As a consequence, men seeking liposuction are mostly concerned with contouring.

The Chin/Neck Area, Abdomen, Flanks and Breast Area

Because the skin of the flanks is generally thick and elastic, liposuction results in a satisfactory shrinkage without losing skin laxity, whereas results in the abdomen/breasts greatly rely on the individual skin quality.[4]

LIPOSUCTION TYPES

Over the decades, liposuction has undergone numerous advances with one common goal: To melt or remove fat and improve the overlying skin's appearance. Since the 1990s, numerous technologies have been developed by exploiting different sources of energy and geared toward ablation and liquefaction of fat to enhance, improve and facilitate traditional liposuction.[5] These include laser-assisted liposuction, water-assisted, radiofrequency (RF)-assisted, and ultrasound-assisted devices.[6] Moreover, because one of the major disadvantages of traditional liposuction is that it has no effect or may in fact worsen skin tightening or cellulite reduction in some anatomic sites such as the abdomen, arms, and inner thighs, these newer devices are hypothesized to improve skin laxity and tone. Power-assisted liposuction is another type of liposuction that was developed with the goal to reduce physician fatigue. Power-assisted liposuction devices use power supplied by an electric motor or compressed air to produce either a rapid in-and-out movement or a spinning rotation of an attached liposuction cannula. The reciprocating action reduces the force needed to perform the liposuction, resulting in a more accurate, gentler, and less traumatic approach. Several physicians prefer to use this type of device to treat men, who have harder and more fibrous tissue than women, and subsequently present greater physical demands on the performing surgeon.[7–9]

Liposuction is performed in the same manner in male patients as it is in females. The most common approach is using the tumescent method, in which a saline solution of lidocaine, epinephrine, and bicarbonate is injected into the area where liposuction is to be performed.[10] The tumescent formula works as a local anesthetic, but also, importantly, it provides hemostasis by constricting the small blood vessels. After infiltration, fat is suctioned using a syringe–cannula, which is connected to an aspirator, into the deep fat layer. The cannula is moved in a back-and-forth motion, and sometimes in cross-hatching manner.[11]

In laser-assisted liposuction, tumescent anesthesia is performed first, after which a 1-mm diameter microcannula encasing a small optical fiber is introduced into the subcutaneous fat. The cannula is passed through the tissues in a back-and-forth motion to achieve an even distribution of laser energy throughout the desired area. Laser settings controlling power and cumulative energy, for example, are determined according to anatomic sites.[12,13] These laser systems stimulate adipocyte burst, thus priming the fat for suctioning. In addition, the laser energy initiates a dermal collagen-tightening response.

In RF-assisted liposuction, delivery of directional RF energy into the subcutaneous fat coagulates and liquefies adipose tissue and gently heats the subcutaneous fibrous matrix and the dermal tissue to subnecrotic contractile levels.

RF-assisted lipoplasty is based on The BodyTite system (Invasix Ltd., Yokneam, Israel), an RF-assisted lipolasty device demonstrated to be safe and effective in the removal of modest volumes of fat while inducing subdermal tissue contraction.[14–17]

Ultrasound-assisted liposuction (UAL) has been developed in 3 forms: external UAL, internal UAL, and vibration amplification of sound energy at resonance.[18,19] External UAL entails transcutaneous application of high-frequency ultrasonic fields delivered into tissue, followed by traditional aspirative liposuction, with the goal of improving the mechanical removal of adipose cells. The use of high-intensity, high-frequency external ultrasound before liposuction has been reported to enhance the ability to extract fat, increase the amount of fat extracted, and decrease patient discomfort during and after liposuction. Internal UAL involves the application of ultrasonic energy through a specialized cannula directly into the subcutaneous tissue followed by traditional aspirative liposuction. In vibration amplification of sound energy at resonance-assisted liposuction, intermittent or continuous bursts of ultrasonic energy is used to break up fat cells, which are then removed by suction.[19,20] Because accumulated fat is denser in male patients, ultrasonic liposuction is a preferable technique to treat male patients.

Water-assisted devices are not that popular in the United States owing to the cost of the device and their lack of effect on skin laxity. Water jet devices use a high-pressure jet of water to separate adipose cells and hydrodissect through tissues while preserving important anatomic structures, thus selectively eliminating fat while sparing blood vessels and nerves.[21–23]

LIPOSUCTION TECHNIQUES ACCORDING TO ANATOMIC AREA
Neck

Neck liposuction is the gold standard to remove a double chin in men. Although not a great amount of fat can be removed, it is enough to create a visible aesthetic difference. With older men, because elasticity is compromised, there may be a need to tighten the loose neck muscles (platysma) via a small, 2-cm incision under the skin. Liposuction can only be performed above the platysma muscles to minimize any complications. Neck liposuction involves marking the area and making an incision at the midline of the neck, 1.25 to 2 inches posterior to the front of the chin, followed by liposuction to the left and right side of the neck. Other practitioners may make an incision behind the ear, but that may result in temporarily affecting the mandible branch of the facial nerve. Although there are currently some noninvasive options to reduce a double chin, such as Kybella[24–27] and Coolscupting using the Cool-mini applicator, a 1-time neck liposuction treatment has been demonstrated to yield consistently good results in only 30 minutes.[28]

Waist and Lower Back

When performing liposuction to these areas, it is recommended to make as few incisions as possible. After placing the patient in the prone position, a small incision (1/4 inches long) is made in the middle of the lower back and suctioning begins to the left and then right side. The patient is then turned to the supine position and 2 small incisions are made in the folds in the groin area at opposite sides of the waist. From these 2 incision points, the rest of the waist and lower back can be suctioned. All incisions sites are closed with 1 suture than can be removed in 5 to 7 days after surgery. Given how fibrous the fat is in this area for men, UAL is a method of choice for many surgeons because it facilitates the liquefying of the tissue, ensuring a smoother contour.[29]

Abdomen

Although the abdomen is a popular location that men request to be reduced via liposuction, it may not be effective to treat conditions like the so-called beer belly. Men have certain amount of fat above the rectus abdominal muscle, but especially in overweight aged men, they have a lot of visceral fat, internally surrounding the organs. Nevertheless, abdominal fat, usually up to one-half of an inch may be liposuctioned with the patient in the supine position through 2 small incisions in the left and right side of the groin. When suctioning the central abdomen, smooth, nonforced, criss-crossing movements are recommended.[29]

Breast

Liposuction is one of the most popular areas to treat a condition in men known as pseudogynecomastia, which does not involve breast tissue but is rather pure fat. This condition often coincides with true gynecomastia, which is enlarged glandular and breast tissue that needs to be removed via excision to bring satisfactory results to the patient. During breast liposuction in men, an incision about one-quarter of an inch long is made between the dark and light part of the areola in each breast, and each breast can be suctioned through each incision as well as the contralateral breast for a more efficient outcome and speedy recovery (**Fig. 1**).[30]

RECOVERY, RISKS, AND COMPLICATIONS

Recovery from liposuction depends on the anatomic area, patient health and compliance with postoperative instructions. On average, recovery from abdominal liposuction is 6 to 12 weeks, for flanks/breasts 8 to 16 weeks, and the neck typically recovers within 6 weeks. Patients will feel sore but can resume their normal activities within 5 days with final results showing within 2 to 3 months. It is recommended to wear a compression garment under their clothing for around 4 weeks postoperatively. Pain, bruising, and swelling are the most common side effects, and over-the-counter nonsteroid any inflammatory drugs are recommended because they will effectively reduce pain and speed up healing.[31–33] In men undergoing abdominal liposuction, it is common to experience genital bruising that lasts around a week after surgery owing to blood and fluids descending as the patient ambulates. These effects spontaneously heal within 1 month. Although often the satisfaction with liposuction outcomes incentivizes patients to maintain results

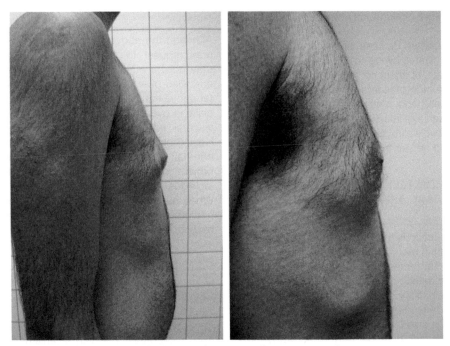

Fig. 1. Before and after liposuction in the breasts. (*Courtesy of* Dr Bruce Katz.)

through a healthy lifestyle with exercise and diet, it is important to stress that weight gain can reverse any positive outcomes. Strenuous exercising is not advised for at least 1 to 2 months after the procedure to allow healing of incisions, but all patients are encouraged to engage in light activity like walking to avoid risk of clotting in their legs (deep venous thrombosis).[34]

Risks of liposuction are fairly low and are essentially the same for both men and women.[35] It is imperative for patients to seek a board-certified plastic surgeon who has 5 years of plastic surgery training after his or her medical training who will perform a thorough consultation to determine whether they are suitable candidates for liposuction. Contraindications include obesity, patients on blood thinners or with coagulopathy, patients with a concomitant infection, patients with severe chronic lymphedema cardiac/pulmonary problems, and patients with any mental health issues; an increasing number of male patients suffer from body dysmorphic disorder.[36] Common side effects after liposuction in men are typically bruising, swelling, and mild irregularities after surgery. Because men have a thicker dermis and do not go through childbirth, irregularities and skin laxity after surgery are less of a concern for them. Complications that can occur include infection, overcorrection, scarring, skin and fat necrosis, fat embolism, deep venous thrombosis, hemorrhage and temporary nerve damage, volume overload, blood loss, loss of sensations, and soft tissue damage.

SUMMARY

Liposuction in men has proven to be a safe, effective way to sculpt the male body and deliver satisfactory outcomes to men of all ethnicities, ages, and cultural backgrounds. The pursuit of beauty in men, manifested in a lean, athletic body with highly defined musculature, can be achieved by traditional and energy-assisted liposuction, sometimes in association with noninvasive fat-reducing options such as cryolipolysis, ultrasound, and acoustic wave therapy. Dermatologic surgeons catering treatments to this population must be sensitive not only to the male anatomy and unique metabolism, but also the distinct behavioral and emotional temperament that men display. Moreover, the paucity of high-level evidence clinical studies on male subjects comparing the various liposuction technologies, techniques, and outcomes needs to be remedied by designing and publishing the relevant research for men.

REFERENCES

1. Surgery, ASfAP, 2016 Cosmetic Surgery National Data Bank Statistics. 2017.
2. Singh B, Keaney T, Rossi AM. Male body contouring. J Drugs Dermatol 2015;14(9):1052–9.

3. Almutairi K, Gusenoff JA, Rubin JP. Body contouring. Plast Reconstr Surg 2016;137(3):586e–602e.
4. Shiffman MA, Giuseppe MASAD. Liposuction principles and practice. In: Shiffman MA, Alberto Di G, MASAD Giuseppe, editors. 2nd edition. Verlag Berlin Heidelberg: Springer; 2016.
5. Flynn TC, Coleman WP 2nd, Field LM, et al. History of liposuction. Dermatol Surg 2000;26(6):515–20.
6. Mann MW, Palm MD, Sengelmann RD. New advances in liposuction technology. Semin Cutan Med Surg 2008;27(1):72–82.
7. Fodor P. Power-assisted lipoplasty. Aesthet Surg J 2001;21(1):90–2.
8. Fodor PB. Power-assisted lipoplasty versus traditional suction-assisted lipoplasty: comparative evaluation and analysis of output. Aesthet Plast Surg 2005;29(2):127.
9. Fodor PB, Vogt PA. Power-assisted lipoplasty (PAL): a clinical pilot study comparing PAL to traditional lipoplasty (TL). Aesthet Plast Surg 1999;23(6):379–85.
10. Lillis PJ. The tumescent technique for liposuction surgery. Dermatol Clin 1990;8(3):439–50.
11. Hanke W, Cox SE, Kuznets N, et al. Tumescent liposuction report performance measurement initiative: national survey results. Dermatol Surg 2004;30(7):967–77 [discussion: 978].
12. Badin AZ, Gondek LB, Garcia MJ, et al. Analysis of laser lipolysis effects on human tissue samples obtained from liposuction. Aesthet Plast Surg 2005;29(4):281–6.
13. Badin AZ, Moraes LM, Gondek L, et al. Laser lipolysis: flaccidity under control. Aesthet Plast Surg 2002;26(5):335–9.
14. Blugerman G, Schavelzon D, Paul MD. A safety and feasibility study of a novel radiofrequency-assisted liposuction technique. Plast Reconstr Surg 2010;125(3):998–1006.
15. Chia CT, Theodorou SJ, Hoyos AE, et al. Radiofrequency-assisted liposuction compared with aggressive superficial, subdermal liposuction of the arms: a bilateral quantitative comparison. Plast Reconstr Surg Glob Open 2015;3(7):e459.
16. Ion L, Raveendran SS, Fu B. Body-contouring with radiofrequency-assisted liposuction. J Plast Surg Hand Surg 2011;45(6):286–93.
17. Keramidas E, Rodopoulou S. Radiofrequency-assisted liposuction for neck and lower face adipodermal remodeling and contouring. Plast Reconstr Surg Glob Open 2016;4(8):e850.
18. Beckenstein MS, Grotting JC. Ultrasound-assisted lipectomy using the solid probe: a retrospective review of 100 consecutive cases. Plast Reconstr Surg 2000;105(6):2161–74 [discussion: 2175–9].
19. de Souza Pinto EB, Abdala PC, Maciel CM, et al. Liposuction and VASER. Clin Plast Surg 2006;33(1):107–15, vii.
20. Hoyos AE, Millard JA. VASER-assisted high-definition liposculpture. Aesthet Surg J 2007;27(6):594–604.
21. Man D, Meyer H. Water jet-assisted lipoplasty. Aesthet Surg J 2007;27(3):342–6.
22. Sasaki GH. Water-assisted liposuction for body contouring and lipoharvesting: safety and efficacy in 41 consecutive patients. Aesthet Surg J 2011;31(1):76–88.
23. Stutz JJ, Krahl D. Water jet-assisted liposuction for patients with lipoedema: histologic and immunohistologic analysis of the aspirates of 30 lipoedema patients. Aesthet Plast Surg 2009;33(2):153–62.
24. Ascher B, Hoffmann K, Walker P, et al. Efficacy, patient-reported outcomes and safety profile of ATX-101 (deoxycholic acid), an injectable drug for the reduction of unwanted submental fat: results from a phase III, randomized, placebo-controlled study. J Eur Acad Dermatol Venereol 2014;28(12):1707–15.
25. Humphrey S, Sykes J, Kantor J, et al. ATX-101 for reduction of submental fat: A phase III randomized controlled trial. J Am Acad Dermatol 2016;75(4):788–97.e7.
26. Jones DH, Carruthers J, Joseph JH, et al. REFINE-1, a multicenter, randomized, double-blind, placebo-controlled, phase 3 trial with ATX-101, an injectable drug for submental fat reduction. Dermatol Surg 2016;42(1):38–49.
27. Rzany B, Griffiths T, Walker P, et al. Reduction of unwanted submental fat with ATX-101 (deoxycholic acid), an adipocytolytic injectable treatment: results from a phase III, randomized, placebo-controlled study. Br J Dermatol 2014;170(2):445–53.
28. Kilmer SL. Prototype CoolCup cryolipolysis applicator with over 40% reduced treatment time demonstrates equivalent safety and efficacy with greater patient preference. Lasers Surg Med 2016;49(1):63–8.
29. Johnson DS, Cook WR Jr. Advanced techniques in liposuction. Semin Cutan Med Surg 1999;18(2):139–48.
30. Maillard GF, Scheflan M, Bussien R. Ultrasonically assisted lipectomy in aesthetic breast surgery. Plast Reconstr Surg 1997;100(1):238–41.
31. Dolsky RL, Newman J, Fetzek JR, et al. Liposuction. History, techniques, and complications. Dermatol Clin 1987;5(2):313–33.
32. Hoefflin SM, Bornstein JB, Gordon M. General anesthesia in an office-based plastic surgical facility: a report on more than 23,000 consecutive office-based procedures under general anesthesia with no significant anesthetic complications. Plast Reconstr Surg 2001;107(1):243–51 [discussion: 252–7].

33. Melvin A. Prevention and treatment of liposuction complications. In: DGA Shiffman MA, Alberto Di G, editors. Liposuction – principles and practice. London: Springer; 2006. p. 777–87.

34. Igra H, Lanzer D. Avoiding complications. In: Hanke CW, Sattler G, editors. Liposuction. 1st ed. Philadelphia: Saunders; 2005. p. 131–40.

35. Hanke CW, Bernstein G, Bullock S. Safety of tumescent liposuction in 15,336 patients. National survey results. Dermatol Surg 1995;21(5):459–62.

36. Glaser DA, Kaminer MS. Body dysmorphic disorder and the liposuction patient. Dermatol Surg 2005;31(5):559–60 [discussion: 561].

Moving?

Make sure your subscription moves with you!

To notify us of your new address, find your **Clinics Account Number** (located on your mailing label above your name), and contact customer service at:

Email: journalscustomerservice-usa@elsevier.com

800-654-2452 (subscribers in the U.S. & Canada)
314-447-8871 (subscribers outside of the U.S. & Canada)

Fax number: 314-447-8029

Elsevier Health Sciences Division
Subscription Customer Service
3251 Riverport Lane
Maryland Heights, MO 63043

*To ensure uninterrupted delivery of your subscription, please notify us at least 4 weeks in advance of move.

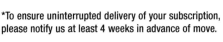

Printed and bound by CPI Group (UK) Ltd, Croydon, CR0 4YY

03/10/2024

01040382-0003